# Because
# YES!

DR. TINA BERNARD

Thank You!
Enjoy the book!
Dr. Tina Bernard 7/28/02

FIRST EDITION

Special Thanks to Kim Renfro for serving to edit this book.

ISBN: 9798811160075

# DEDICATION

This book is dedicated to my husband, Jason, and our children, Holidae, Danielle, and Taylin. Thank you for teaching me to say YES! through your incredible bravery and the power of story.

# CONTENTS

# CHAPTER ONE

## HUMBLE BEGINNINGS

I cannot promise all the stories you are about to read are completely true, but they are my truth as best remembered. The funny part of life is that it really is about your version of reality. Every single day you get to choose what you believe is true. I choose to believe what I post on Facebook for my friends and family to read is truth. My super smart and gorgeous kids are involved in a zillion extracurricular activities, we go on lots of adventures as a family, and I love to post about silly things- like the time I found a pacifier in the toilet. The messy details of the daily grind that beat you down and make you question every fiber of your being are purposefully omitted. Nobody needs to know that my husband leaves his underwear by the toilet every morning despite my ineffectual attempts to change his behavior. And that, my friends, is the essence of YES!

I have tried writing different versions of this book for years. The question for me was always, "Who will want to read this?" Well, the truth is I am authoring this book for myself while hoping to inspire you to understand that life is not exactly what we see on the Hallmark Channel. The plot is not always, "First comes love, then comes marriage, then comes you pushing a baby carriage." Oftentimes, our version of reality is what we live, experience, and how we respond to real life; the life that happens when the dishwasher and washing machine go out in the same week, your kids are sick, your spouse is out of town, and you have no idea when you last showered.

This is the honest-to-goodness truth about a real-life, small-town girl who grew up across the street from the cornfields. In my little hometown, we paid no attention to silos, rusty old milk jugs, or the stuff my grandma saved in case she needed it someday. This part of the story will come full circle in subsequent chapters, but the truth is that life was simple. It was a big deal when our little town got a blinking red light. It was comical to give directions because there was nothing to reference. You couldn't even say, "Take a left at the Dairy Queen," because the nearest Dairy Queen was a good 30-minute drive away.

The same was true for groceries. You had to drive for about 20-30 minutes to buy milk. If you had a midnight craving for ice cream, it was an hour-long road trip. Just as driving long distances for groceries was our normal, so was the short distance to a cold beer. If you wanted a beer, all you had to do was go next door, around the block, or down the road to grab a cold one from a neighbor. Everyone had plenty of beer and whiskey. My dad, her dad, his dad, their dad, all the dads had an open bar ready for you to stop by. The only rule back then was that if you wanted a beer, you had to stay and drink it. This ultimately led to more beer, which then led us to the pasture, turned into an all-night party, and resulted in lots of stories and fun. Man, we had some fun!

One thing that I remember is that nobody really worried about drinking ages, but everyone seemed to care about driving. In my hometown, we didn't drive once we started drinking. The assumption was that you were spending the night wherever you were if you took even one sip. If we accidentally found ourselves in a pasture, there was usually a bonfire involved. The local sheriff would follow the smoke and offer us a ride home. Sometimes our parents were with us; sometimes they weren't. It didn't matter; we just never drove.

My upbringing is essential to the story because it defines a humble beginning, in a small Texas town, with a family that was nothing short of *Leave it to Beaver*. My parents are still married, as were my grandparents. My dad served as a deacon in our Baptist church, and my parents led the youth group's Sunday School lessons. I know, I know. Baptists aren't supposed to drink or dance. We did both; we just didn't talk about it at church.

When I was little, my parents took a continuing education course to learn sign language because they wanted to communicate better with my dad's best friend, Larry. It was a 45-minute drive to the community college, but they called it "Date Night." My mom enjoyed the courses and discovered a passion for signing. She went on to earn her associate degree as an interpreter for the deaf within a few years. I remember my family making a big deal about my mom's graduation. That was my first experience with success in the academic world. I remember the pictures we took of her and the pride in my grandparents' eyes. She had done what no other member of her family had done, and it was inspiring.

We lived the All-American dream. We were small-town, but we knew how to work hard, love deeply, and come together to help a neighbor. These values are ingrained in me as deeply as the idea that if you aren't 15 minutes early, you are late. The truths that define us are subject to what we have experienced and the context in which we have experienced them. Our past is to be understood, but it does not dictate where our future leads. While I have an almost picture-perfect upbringing, there are lessons that I have learned along the way that help me understand the importance of respecting what has been, so that whatever is next is my choice. As it is yours. Because YES!

# CHAPTER TWO

## MILK

Milk is a theme that runs throughout my life story. The first story describes the birth of my first child and the moment the milk came in. It was the first time in my life I realized people don't talk about the hard stuff. Not one person in my life told me about what happens to our bodies after we have a baby. I remember feeling angry at every other woman who had a baby and failed to tell me what happened next. The second time milk enters the story is when we found out our middle child not only had a swallowing dysfunction but was also allergic to milk. I learned that our bodies are a mystery, and doctors don't always have the answers. The most recent milk episode deals with my understanding of human behaviors and how easily our world manipulates our thinking. When I presented my dissertation research, I used the placement of milk in a grocery store to represent the idea of "You don't know what you don't know!" It is interesting to note the irony of milk playing such a huge role in developing this book. The YESisms are a direct result of understanding the interconnectedness of my experiences and surrendering to His purpose for my life. Because YES!

I don't remember much about the birth of my first child because it was a horrendous experience. My husband and I were at the doctor's office when my blood pressure and pre-eclampsia became so out of control that my daughter, Holidae, was delivered two weeks early. She and I went into cardiac arrest and faced death straight in the face. Thankfully, she came out perfect and was just fine. I, on the other hand, had some complications. After two days of sedation, I was just waking up when my milk came in. You guys. Nobody told me about the milk. I remember being so upset when this happened. The milk came flooding in and swelled my boobs to the point where I had to carry them with both hands. The nurse came in and tried to stick my newborn baby on my raw nipples, and I about lost it. I had no idea what to do or how to deal with these new boulders. From then on, anytime my daughter would cry, my milk would soak through the pads, and my shirt would be so wet, you could ring it out. I had milk fill the nodules in my underarms. I found myself crying in the shower, wondering why nobody ever told me about the horror of milk boobs. I made a vow almost two decades ago to never hide this part of motherhood from anyone. From that moment, I realized that the only way we can help each other is to talk about the hard stuff, like milk boobs.

The other thing that no one told me about was the loneliness that comes with just giving birth. I mean, I thought it would be great to have a baby and take six weeks off from work. But for a total people person, this was the loneliest period of my life. Let me explain. In my world, people have their moms stay with them the first week after a new baby arrives. That was my expectation but didn't turn out to be my truth.

My mom had already been with us for ten days before the baby came because my stupid dog split himself in half. Shadow, our 11-month-old Labrador Retriever, was focused on a kid on a bicycle rather than the stationary fence post. The dog turned too quickly, crashed into the pole, and bust open his mid-section in half. His injuries required surgery and stitches. Since I was on bed rest, my mom had to come to stay with us and babysit the dadgum dog. She had used her vacation days to help us before the baby even arrived.

My husband took off for a week after our daughter was born. His spring break allowed for one week to become two full weeks. I thought he would help me with the baby, the dishes, laundry, something. Instead, he put in a garden and mowed the lawn. I say this with all the love in the world… guys just don't know. Instead of having one baby, I felt that I was now taking care of the three of us. Alone.

By the time my mom came back to help, I was three weeks postpartum, and I was a wreck. My milk boobs were humongous, I was exhausted, and now my precious daughter only wanted her daddy. To complicate things, the new aforementioned garden needed to be watered. I knew that if I wanted to experience any bit of happiness in this new role, I would have to dig deep inside and find joy despite my newfound responsibilities and expectations.

We survived. I remember my glorious first days back to work. Everyone kept saying, "Are you okay?" YES~!! I was better than ever! Finally, somebody else was dealing with my infant, and I got to be back in the world of people. Thank God. This was when I learned there are people called to take care of infants. Unfortunately, I am not one of those people. I do not look at sweet little baby pictures and think, "Oh, how precious! What a bundle of joy!" I mean, I love baby toes, but holding an infant does nothing for me. The thought of being responsible for a tiny human terrifies me.

Much of my testimony revolves around the lessons learned as a mom. Motherhood didn't start with rainbows and sunshine. My husband and I met in May and married in July. It was a crazy, whirlwind beginning, and like most things in our life, it began on a whim. My mom was planning a birthday party for my nephew on July 27th. I joked and said, "Well, we were going to get married that day." My husband went along with the "joke," and we decided at that moment to spend the rest of our lives together. We literally hadn't gone on a real adult date when we decided to marry. It's the truth, and almost two decades later, I suppose the joke is still going strong.

Our oldest daughter was a few months old when she developed an infection in her bloodstream. For weeks, I screamed something was wrong with her, but nobody could figure out what was going on. She was prescribed antibiotic after antibiotic until one day, her fever went up to 105, and she was lethargic. Despite our best efforts, nothing was working. We found a new doctor's office open on a Sunday morning, and I was the first one in line. The receptionist said there were no appointments, so I planted myself in the waiting room, hysterically crying, and demanded someone help us. It was ridiculous, but guess what? That morning, she received an injection of a high-powered antibiotic called Rocephin (probably to appease me), and the doctor sent us for X-rays and bloodwork. By 11 p.m., the doctor called and said, "Your daughter is septic. I'm meeting you at the hospital. Do I need to send an ambulance?" Um. No. We threw our shoes on and flew to the hospital, praying the whole time. It turns out our baby daughter had a pneumococcal infection and was treated with IV antibiotics.

We spent nine days in the hospital that time. Unfortunately, that story didn't end there. Two weeks later, our daughter was readmitted to the hospital with the same symptoms but greater severity. It was awful. We spent almost a month in the hospital, and a specialist was brought in from out of state to investigate how the infection came back so violently. Apparently, this was highly uncommon and complicated. The medical staff ordered countless tests and diagnostic procedures. The worst test was a 24-hour HIV/AIDS test. Remember that my husband and I only dated for around nine weeks before marrying. We were not each other's firsts, so I looked at him, and he looked at me. We knew that if she had HIV/AIDS, we all did. Our entire family unit was at stake, and the impending perception of doom flooded through our veins. Thankfully, HIV/AIDS was not our reality. I remember feeling so vividly that our choices in life all have consequences. At that moment, I wondered if my carefree past had finally caught up with me. To this day, her illness is still unexplained. We do not have answers, but I learned a lesson about life being precious.

Without realizing it, I had forgotten all about the pain and discomfort of my dreadfully painful milk boobs and the early misperceived loneliness. The seriousness of the illness our daughter faced overshadowed all previous feelings of discontent with the circumstances of the present. I began to wonder if people don't talk about the hard stuff because they forget just how hard it is. Maybe something harder happens. Maybe it is just easier to forget. Either way, I think it is important to honor where we have been, share our stories with others, and encourage one another to talk about the hard stuff. Because YES!

.

# CHAPTER THREE

# THE LOST TOE

The next time we faced jaw-dropping defeat occurred when our second daughter, Dani, was born. Like her big sister, she was born two weeks early due to my pre-eclampsia issues. That girl was on fire from the moment she came out of the womb. She was and has always been strong and mighty! I was excited about the opportunity for a do-over since my first experience with Motherhood was full of trauma. Well, the second verse was the same as the first.

My daughter hated me worse than the first one. She cried all the time. This girl kept me up all day, all night, all the time. She would calm down occasionally with her dad, and I remember understanding why some species eat their young. The post-partum depression with this kid was quintessentially the worst. To make matters worse, she wouldn't stop crying!

One night, she was utterly inconsolable. I mean, cry, cry, cry. The only thing that helped was to hold her like an NFL running back would cradle a football. I would bend over, tuck her under my arm, swing her back, and pull her up swiftly. This went on for hours, and I remember being completely exhausted. I had just started back to work and felt incredibly guilty about missing another day. I also felt it was my responsibility to stay up all night trying to keep this little monster quiet so my husband would get a good night's sleep. But, by 4 a.m. on this night, I decided that enough was enough. I was taking her to the ER. I told my husband that he had to figure out how to get our other kid to daycare.

I began getting my baby ready, and her toe fell off. TRUE STORY! I took off her footed pajamas, and my baby's second left toe fell off in my hand. A Barbie's hair had wrapped around the end of her toe and cut off the circulation. I have absolutely no idea how a Barbie's hair was in the bottom of the pajamas, but I am guessing it had something to do with the laundry. My baby had been crying because her toe wasn't getting blood. The football hold and swinging action forced blood down to her feet, which made her feel better. Other than that, she was in pain and losing a toe. No wonder she was crying! OMG! I threw the toe into a bag with milk (because that is what you do- right?), grabbed the baby, jumped into the car, and drove like a maniac to the hospital. The emergency room physician put salve and a band-aid on the toe and sent us home. It was fine. She was fine. The toe grew back, and none of my kids wore footed pajamas again.

Unfortunately, that was only the beginning of health issues for that kid. She was sick pretty much from birth on. She was born in early November, and by Christmas, I was exhausted. She cried all the time, even when her toe was better. We thought she had colic, so we tried different formulas. On Christmas Eve, she had a little cough, but I was so tired that I didn't realize how bad her cough had gotten. We were at my parent's house (across from the cornfields) when my mom volunteered to stay up on Christmas night with her. The next morning, I woke up to an eerie sound. My daughter was not crying. I went into the living room to check on her, and her lips were light blue. I tried to shake her and wake her up, but she was just lifeless, and the more I tried to arouse her, the more I realized she was not breathing as she should.

We didn't have time to wait for an ambulance. My husband began driving to the hospital while I performed CPR on my 7-week-old infant in the back of our minivan. My mom called 911, and the local sheriff was soon behind us, providing a police escort to the hospital. I yelled at my husband to GO! despite the police presence. I tried explaining the necessity for speed while focusing on two fingers just above the tiny chest and forcing small puffs of air into my daughter's lungs. I was agitated that my husband didn't understand this element of small-town emergencies. What didn't he understand? We were not being pulled over; we were being escorted! When we arrived at the hospital, the medical staff was ready for us and took my lifeless infant away. I ran in but had to wait in the ER waiting room while the doctors and nurses stabilized her. After what seemed like an eternity, the medical team had her stable and on oxygen. Thank GOD!

That afternoon, we were transferred to an ICU unit in a large children's hospital closer to our home. Our local children's hospital sent an ambulance for us. I sat helpless in the front of the ambulance while my daughter coded twice. I cannot explain to you how that feels, but I'll never forget the words, "We're losing her." My husband was following the ambulance, and I remember being so thankful that he was nearby yet so angry that he wasn't with me. It was an out-of-body experience that I pray no other parent must endure.

That episode had a happy ending in that our daughter was diagnosed with RSV and recovered within a few weeks. Kind of. I mean, her symptoms improved, but she was still crying constantly and never really seemed well. We kept blaming RSV for the newly acquired asthma and long-term antibiotics. The problem was that she kept getting sick. This is when I learned the value of data collection and keeping good records. I kept a calendar of medications, doctor's visits, temperatures, etc... The records helped me determine that every single time my baby had an antibiotic, there was a period of improvement followed by fever within 24 hours of stopping the antibiotic. I recorded data and searched for answers. I showed our pediatrician the data and sought out specialists, getting second and third opinions.

Finally, I found a team in Houston, Texas, that specialized in lung functioning. One doctor on the team ordered a swallow dysfunction study which literally took less than 20 minutes. The test showed our daughter was aspirating on thin liquids. This entire time, every illness was a direct result of a swallowing dysfunction. How do you fix that? My baby was prescribed a substance called "Thick It" which is a powder that changes thin liquids into thicker consistencies. Her body was able to retrain itself to swallow correctly within weeks of starting this substance, and she began to heal. Thank GOD. To this day, she still has damage to her lungs and residual asthma issues from months of a swallowing dysfunction that resulted in her aspirating on thin liquids, but for the most part, she was better.

The experience with the toe falling off was a weird, bizarre, yet relatively common problem with an easy solution. I couldn't see what was going on until I totally took off all layers and really looked at her closely. Both the toe and swallowing dysfunction leads me to beg any of you fighting health issues to find what is causing the problem. What is the problem at the core? How can YOU take ownership of the root cause? Who can help you? If you feel that your doctor isn't listening, it is your responsibility to find someone who will. You are the boss. Because YES!

.

# CHAPTER FOUR

## ELVIS AND A NEW CHURCH HOME

Once the dust settled from the second daughter, Dani, things seemed to normalize. Of course, I was ecstatic with my little family and our life. We were excited about the future. Two years before Dani was born, my husband and I had started our master's degrees. We both graduated the summer after she was born. Additionally, we celebrated five years of marriage and my 30th birthday that summer. An Elvis impersonator and about 200 of our closest family members and friends joined us in a glorious celebration. It was fun, funky, and downright hilarious. I mean, how can someone forget dentures flying across the table while Elvis sings, "Hunka Hunka Burning Love!"

Oh, how fun! Until my mom ended the evening because my grandfather had taken a turn for the worse. The next day, we took my grandpa off life support, fully intending for him to take his last breath while we were gathered as a family. Nope. That's not how that worked. I mean, I guess it can, but that was not our experience. It took five days for him to die. I know, I know. That sounds horrible. But it was the worst five days of my life up until that point. Life became a ridiculous waiting game. I finally crafted a plan to have my aunt flown in, mostly because my mom was a wreck and needed her sister. The day after she got there, my grandpa gave it up. I think he was waiting for her. I was so thankful that it was over and that my aunt was here. We needed her. He needed her. My mom needed her. Thank GOD.

This was the first real experience I had with death. I mean, we had known people who had died, but no one had been close to us. My grandpa was the patriarch of the family. I had no idea, really, about family secrets until that point. Come to find out, my grandpa had been married previously and had two other kids somewhere in New York. Wow. I had no idea. My grandparent's marriage was not exactly picture-perfect as I thought it had been all my life. I suppose this may have been the first time I realized just how sheltered I had been from reality. I mean, my grandpa was a great guy. He loved us. He loved his family. He sacrificed for his country as a Navy man. But the man that I put on a pedestal wasn't perfect. I've come to understand more about the choices in his life, but this taught me that things aren't always as they seem.

Not much time passed after my grandpa's death before my mother-in-law, Linda, became sick. Her health deteriorated rather quickly because of heart damage and disease. She was a woman of great integrity and commitment. She and my father-in-law had been married longer than my parents. My husband and I come from a long line of committed marriages that were only separated by death. Linda died before my third child was born.

My husband's family has a way of thinking optimistically about the future, no matter how bleak the prognosis might be. I wish I had that ability. Instead, I tend to deal with things head-on and in the moment. I tried to warn them that Linda was very sick and on her death bed, but the reality of the situation was too unbearable for most of the family to accept. My mother-in-law passed away with her family surrounding her at the hospital and I'll never forget the beautiful quilt draped over her body as she passed by the waiting room. The events that transpired afterward were unbelievable.

The day after Linda died, the family met at the funeral home to make arrangements. Fortunately, the family had purchased plots in a nearby cemetery. Unfortunately, there was no money for a service or casket. The family agreed to cremate the body and host a private service at a later date, but for now, there was a plan. The only place big enough for everyone to gather was an abandoned, empty house one of the uncles had purchased. I went over to the house with my husband to make a plan for a memorial service, and he began to weep, declaring, "My mom deserves more than this." I couldn't have agreed more.

That night, I began to pray more than I had in a long time. I grew up in the Baptist Church. I knew God. I was baptized. I was saved. My

13

husband and I were married in a church, and we had taken our kids to church a few times. But I hadn't really been cognizant of God's presence in recent years. I knew, though, that churches had sanctuaries and kitchens. My experience was that when a person died, a service was held at a church, followed by a family meal. I didn't have a church home, but I knew Church was home. The next day, I woke up and went to church.

Random. It was totally random. I went on a Friday morning, and there was only a handful of people there. Many churches are closed on Fridays, but this one morning, a special pastor was there. He welcomed me into his office, and we prayed. He offered to do a service without charge in their church that Sunday afternoon. Y'all. It was perfect. God totally opened that door, and I believe it changed our family all for the better. It gave our family a plan and a decent place to say our goodbyes to Linda. We still had the "reception" at the abandoned house, but it gave us a few days to clean and get things together. The family met at the church, we had a respectful service, and we gathered in a home. My friends stepped up and served my husband's family. My family went out of their way to do things for my in-laws, and it all worked out. I have no doubt in my mind that it was explicitly God's plan to bring us to the church we still call home. Because YES!

# CHAPTER FIVE

## HERNIAS, SURGERIES, AND COLD FEET

By this point, you've read about two of my kids' births and a few of their illnesses. You've also read about two deaths. Geesh! Welcome to my life! I could go on and on about various random illnesses that the kids faced, or the time when I got a staph infection on my panty line and required home health to pack the wound, or when I had my wisdom teeth become locked-jaw for almost a month, or when Holly's arm became dislodged from trying to get her out of the dog food, but let's not. I mean, someday, I can let you buy me a drink, and we can swap stories, but let's continue.

Every four years, my mom's side of the family gathers in Missouri for a family reunion. In the summer of 2012, I invited my grandmother on a pre-family reunion adventure. I took my grandma, both my daughters, and my niece and nephew to the Oklahoma Zoo. Jason couldn't join us because he was working. So, it was me, grandma, and four kids. We had a great time at the zoo, grabbed some pizza afterward, then went back to the hotel to swim. I remember getting a six-pack of beer to drink, and I couldn't even finish one without feeling nauseous. I should have known something was up. The next day, we arrived in Missouri and met up with the rest of the family for the reunion. My grandma was the baby of nine children, so there were a ton of aunts, uncles, and cousins. We had the best time catching up, playing cards, and singing old country songs while the cousins picked their guitars.

My extended family makes moonshine. I love the apple-pie moonshine, but the minute it touched my lips on this trip, I started puking. Suddenly, a previous conversation in which my cousin Tiffany declared how much she wanted another baby started playing in my mind. Then, I recalled how in the pool in Oklahoma, the beer didn't taste good. My new Victoria's Secret bras were hurting me. The entire drive home from Missouri (through all the hills), I felt sick. When we arrived home, I bought a pregnancy test. It obviously was not the Victoria's Secret bras that made my boobs sore.

I texted my husband, "Please bring home a strawberry milkshake." He immediately texted back, "You better not be pregnant." Um. Well. The only time in my life I had ever craved strawberry milkshakes was when I was pregnant. I don't really even like milkshakes or strawberries for that matter. So, by the time he got home, he had already figured out what I was about to tell him. He asked, "How do you come home pregnant from a family reunion?" Ha! True story. I totally came home pregnant... of course, I left home pregnant, but I didn't know it. I mean, it was not even on our radar because we had tried for a few years unsuccessfully to have another baby and had basically given up.

After our middle child was born, we had a miscarriage. I was devastated. We were barely pregnant, but we were indeed pregnant. I didn't even make it to my first appointment, but I felt the loss. I know, I know... it's a thing. But for me, it was real. I still wonder what happened or why, but it didn't seem to matter to anyone else. It came and went. I think about him/ her often, but I'm probably the only person who does. My husband had only about six days of knowing about the pregnancy before it was over. I don't blame him; I just understand where some women are coming from when they talk about the loss of an unborn child. It was a part of me that I'd never get to meet or know.

Nonetheless, I had come home from the family reunion pregnant. This time, it felt real. I made a doctor's appointment, and sure enough, it was real. In fact, we were already nine weeks pregnant! I couldn't believe it. I threw up daily when I was pregnant with the girls. I remember the doctor asking me if I wanted genetic testing since I was "older." Ha! NO. I mean, yes. I mean, I don't know. No. We didn't want to know anything except for the baby's sex.

I remember that appointment like it was yesterday. Jason and I were in the room, and the doctor asked if we wanted to know. YES! He said it was a boy and I didn't believe him. I made the doctor circle the penis and printed out the picture from the screen. I wanted a boy my entire life. I mean, someone to go fishing with, dance with me, and do boy things. YAY!! A real-live boy. And even weirder, I had a penis growing inside me! What?? That was C-R-A-Z-Y! I still get giddy when I think about that day. We went straight to Babies-R-Us and bought everything BOY. Footballs, baseballs, fishing, etc… if it was boy-related, we bought it! Yay!!

Then, I should have known. Things seemed to get weirder by the minute. The baby's original due date was around Valentine's Day. I was put on bedrest the Friday before Thanksgiving due to pre-eclampsia. That was normal, though, for me. I knew he'd be delivered two weeks early via C-section. My husband and I joked about how cool it would be if the baby shared a birthday with the king of Rock-n-Roll. We had no idea that on January 8th (Elvis's birthday), my water would break. My water never broke during the pregnancies with the girls, so I thought I had peed myself in the middle of a mid-morning nap. I woke up, and the wetness continued. Upon some internet surfing, I learned that the PH balance in amniotic fluid was different from pee. So, I peed in a cup and compared it to the leaking fluid using a pool test strip. Most certainly, there was a difference in the PH balance between the two liquids, so I headed to the hospital. I didn't tell anyone because it was a little embarrassing to have tested myself with a pool test strip, but the doctors confirmed my water broke and we were having a baby. I called my husband. He was so in shock that his first words were, "What do you want me to do about it?" Ha! GET HERE!~

And so it began. We had a baby that afternoon, and although he was six weeks early, he was perfect and strong- just super little. I remember the first time I saw him; he looked transparent. He was so little. Four little pounds of love. I felt great! I had a great, almost perfect day. My pastor was there, my parents, my husband, our kids, etc… everyone! The doctor came in and asked everyone to leave except my husband. That's when I knew. My heart fell into my stomach as the doctor said, "He's got a little hole in his back. It doesn't appear to be leaking spinal fluid at this time, but you'll need to follow up as soon as possible with your pediatrician. It could be Spina

Bifida." Our lives changed forever that day. Our pastor was the first one back in the room. I remember the look on Brother Jerry's face as he said, "We're just going to give that to God." We prayed.

Then, I did what all moms do. I Googled "Hole in the back" and "Spina Bifida." I honestly do not know what happened next. I know that my milk came in again, like it had after the last two births, and I know that I bled crazy bad again. I remember my son needing light therapy because he was a bit jaundiced. I remember he was itty, bitty tiny. I remember that in one of his first pictures, he was smaller than a regulation football. I remember he was smaller than a loaf of bread and that his feet were the size of a peppermint. I remember feeling completely helpless.

The worry did not subside, even with the first doctor's visit. There were no outward concerns, just a hole in his back. We were referred to a specialist, and then the strangest thing happened. I was changing his diaper, and all of a sudden, these things popped out. I screamed so loudly, and my husband came running in. There were two giant knots popping out on each side of his groin. It was awful. I thought for sure he was hemorrhaging or something. So, I raced him to the ER. Jason had to stay home with the girls, but I had to get to help, fast! I don't even know how my car got parked, but I ran in with my baby, crying hysterically. I tried to explain what was happening, but apparently, I was so ridiculous that they took me straight back. Quickly a nurse was there, and I tried to show her what was going on, but when they took off my son's diaper, the knots were gone. GONE! What??!! I was beside myself. I just knew they were about to admit ME! I called my husband (completely hysterical), and just as quickly as the knots had disappeared, they reappeared. I screamed for a doctor, and she came running in. Looking back on it now, it must have been hilarious to watch me because the doctor simply massaged the knots right back into place. They were hernias. My son had hernias popping out, and they did need surgery to fix them, but it was not an emergency. I, on the other hand, had to have oxygen. No lie. So, off we went and the next day, we met with a surgeon. Good Lord.

Now, the good thing is that our son needed surgery. At this point, the doctors were unable to know exactly how bad the Spina Bifida was because my son was too little to be put under for a CT scan or MRI. But now that he had to have surgery, we were able to schedule a battery of tests that included a CT scan. The doctors also discovered a heart murmur just before surgery. This was a blessing and a curse. The surgery was delayed while they tested the heart. Thankfully, the surgery was back on within a few hours.

The next few days were filled with bad news. Every. Single. Time. A specialist walked into the room, there was a new, more bleak diagnosis and prognosis. Our son had confirmed Spina Bifida, Tethered Cord Syndrome, Lipomas on his spine, neurogenic bowels, neurogenic bladder, and three congenital heart defects. Then, he developed the same bloodstream infection that Holly had when she was a baby, and we were in the hospital for weeks. It was awful. I was still on maternity leave, but Jason had to go back to work during the day. I was alone. All alone. With huge boobs, a terribly sick baby, two little girls to coordinate, and every diagnosis under the sun to Google. And my feet were cold. I don't know why it is so cold in a hospital, but my feet were always cold. Because YES!

# CHAPTER SIX

## THE PROSTHETICS CLINIC

One thing I have learned about medicine is that you deal with one thing at a time. You address the most threatening problem first and work backward. While we were in the hospital for our son's hernias, the doctors found systemic problems throughout his body. He developed an infection after the surgery, which extended our stay. The infection trumped everything because we had to keep the kid alive before we could even think about anything else. So, hernia, then infection, then go home. What? Yes. The hernia doctors do not treat spina bifida. The infection doctors do not treat anything but infection. We had to coordinate the next levels of care outside the perimeter of the hospital- on our own. By we, I mean me. I had to figure out what was next with two little girls, an infant, and huge boobs. And loneliness. So much loneliness. Our extended family was there for us, but they didn't know how to help. My husband was right by my side, but not really. He had to work. Instead of having a sweet eight-week maternity leave to bond with my baby, I spent every single second worrying, scheduling appointments, and having diagnosis after diagnosis handed to me.

I spent countless hours figuring out how to make things happen. I was finally able to go back to teaching at a local elementary school when our son was 15 weeks old, but only for about a week before his next surgery was scheduled. I worked for about three weeks before taking a leave of absence for the remainder of the school year. We thought I could go back to work in the Fall. That didn't happen. I tried. I worked for two weeks before our son spiked a high fever which landed him in the hospital for another two days. I resigned from my teaching position the day after Labor Day. I hadn't worked since the Thanksgiving break of the previous school year, and our savings were gone. Times were hard, but there was no choice but to become a full-time stay-at-home mom. I wasn't sure how we would eat, but I knew that I couldn't continue working and caring for my special needs child. The first days after resigning were full of calls to insurance companies, programs for special needs kids, etc. We made too much money to qualify for food stamps or WIC, and you had to apply to be eligible for anything else. I had to go to the welfare department for an interview to receive Medicaid. We didn't qualify. But, we did qualify for free medical insurance for the kids through CHIPS. That was a blessing. We also qualified for the Children with Special Health Care Needs program. The catch was that the CSHCN program had a three-year waiting period. Good Lord. The benefit to having a child with neurogenic bowels and bladder was the doctors were able to prescribe diapers, and CHIPS covered them. That was helpful.

Another thing that was helpful was Early Childhood Intervention (ECI) services. A caseworker came to our home once a week. She coordinated weekly physical therapy, nutritional consults, home health, and even offered to provide monthly childcare services so we could get groceries or whatever was needed. Every single day for three years, there was a professional in my home, helping my child (unless we were in the hospital).

And, boy, we were in the hospital often. Our son had more tests, more procedures, and more pokes than any child should ever endure. I still have a note from one of the doctors explaining to me that we should join a support group because our son would never sit, stand, or walk. In the note, he calls me out with something like, "Mom is having a hard time coming to an understanding of the prognosis." Whatever. I absolutely was, but it was rude for him to write that. I never liked being in the hospital or hearing bad news. Ever. For that doctor to write that I was having a hard time was unnecessary. I think all parents struggle with coming to terms with the challenges our kids face. I decided, though, to try and connect with other families that had kids with disabilities. There was one occasion when they had a

"Disability Day" at a local waterpark. I had no idea what to expect, and what I witnessed took me totally by surprise. There were lots of kids in wheelchairs that would roll up to the pool and then walk in. What? How was that even possible? I found out that wheelchairs aren't always indicative of the ability to walk. Rather, the ability to walk long distances and stay upright for extended periods of time. It was interesting and enlightening. To be honest, it was also very overwhelming.

On many occasions, our family stayed at the Ronald McDonald House in Austin, Texas. The children's hospital in Austin offers a team approach to treating kids with Spina Bifida. The philosophy is each person on the team is involved in the action care plan for your child. When you go to the clinic, you see all the people- all the doctors- and they work together to make a plan. Instead of a piecemeal approach we were trying to navigate, the team approach in Austin worked well for us. Our son, Taylin, stayed with them until our insurance ran out and we had to transfer to Scottish Rite Hospital in Dallas, Texas. Well, that turned out to also be a blessing because they, too, take a team approach. The only thing we were apprehensive about at Scottish Rite Hospital is that they do not deal with heart conditions. That meant we had to find a cardiologist in the D/FW metroplex and try to incorporate them into the action plan.

The good thing was that we knew about the heart defects, but they weren't affecting our son's quality of life or causing any kind of systemic problems. In medicine, if it isn't broken, you don't really fix it. So, we waited. Surgeries, procedures, and tests continued every three months for almost four years. During one of the visits to Scottish Rite, it was determined that our son needed braces to help him stand. We went to a prosthetics clinic to have specialty braces fitted for his feet and ankles. That was one of the most humbling experiences possible. If you ever need a piece of humble pie, go sit in a prosthetics clinic. It will change you. I remember a sign on the wall that said, "I'm Possible." Instead of impossible, it was a totally different message. I remembered the Bible verse, "I can do all things through Him who gives me strength." Although I knew that the braces on my son's feet offered hope for him to learn to stand and walk, I knew that I, too, was learning to walk by faith. Because YES!

# CHAPTER SEVEN

## IMA PICKER

I began teaching for the University of Phoenix four years before Taylin was born. Even though I had to resign from working full time in a local school district, I was able to continue working for the university online. The problem was that courses are determined by student enrollment and adjunct professors, like me, were not guaranteed consistent work. Thus, I had to figure out a way to supplement our income. In college, I cleaned houses and did my fair share of babysitting, but this was different. I could not leave my infant, nor could I host other kids in my home. Instead, the Lord provided a much different way to earn money than I could ever have imagined.

All the late nights I spent awake, holding a fussy baby were about to come to fruition. The show, American Pickers, caught my attention. The premise is that these two guys travel around, digging through people's junk and find "treasures" that other people buy. The junk they purchased looked old and dusty, but what intrigued me was the fascination with history that is portrayed in the show. These pickers liked to focus on vintage motorcycles. I have no desire to know or learn anything about motorcycles, but I knew that I could learn about vintage items. I began to dabble into the world of picking. I could probably write an entire book about "Pickin' and a Grinnin!" but for now, I'll just highlight some of the wackiest moments.

I started off at garage and estate sales. I cleaned out my own barn and purchased a couple of things that I thought looked cool, then I had my own sale. I made money. I made a couple of hundred dollars off junk. I took that money and bought some more junk. The only real rule I had was to not lose money. I studied junk and people. The fascination with junk intrigued me and I began to study how humans behave when they connect to material things. Some people love the thrill of a good deal. Some people love the memories. Some people believe in the projected value that an item may hold. For me, it was just junk and a way to make money to feed my family. This money was cash, and I could earn as much as I wanted to invest. It was fabulous. So, I threw myself into the research and began making bigger purchases and making more money.

There was also a show called, "Storage Wars" where people purchase storage units. These storage units were left unpaid and unattended by their original purchasers for many reasons. The weird part was that people would bid on a huge storage unit full of boxes that had been left unattended for months. The bidder had no idea about what was in the boxes, so it was very much like gambling. The show highlights rare gems found in boxes and boxes full of junk. Sometimes the investment pays off. Other times, it was boxes full of junk. However, the pickin' and the storage building worlds were about to collide with my world.

I had earned three thousand dollars within the first two months. I wasn't by any means rich, but I was holding my own, making smart buys, and shocking the heck out of my family and friends. Mostly, I was driving my husband crazy. He hates junk and our home looking junky. Our yard was becoming cluttered, and he was going insane. That's when I received the weirdest call of all. A lady, desperate for cash, offered to sell me two storage units and three full barns full of junk for $1,200. She said, "Lady, if you can't make $10,000 off of this stuff, you are terrible at this." Game On. I went and peeked at it, paid her the money, and she told me I had 24 hours to get it all out. 24 hours? I had an infant and a minivan. There were essentially five storage units full of junk to get out in 24 hours!! Yikes!! Did I mention that I hadn't told my husband what I had done?

I had met some pickin' buddies along the way. I knew one guy that worked for another guy and where he lived, so I drove straight over to his house. I asked him to work for me for 24 hours. He grabbed his keys and trailer and followed me over to the units. He and his girlfriend made trip after trip from the units to my house. By this time, we had junk everywhere. There was junk in the front yard, back yard, barns, under the patio, and in our house. That's when my husband got home from work. It was as though World War III began. He was so mad! It was a Monday night and Jason was overwhelmed by the floor to ceiling, all over the yard, undeniable mess that I had gotten myself into. Oy Vey!

The two experienced pickers helped me set up as much of the large items as we could in the front yard. We began the first ever "Pickin' Party" on Thursday. We just started making up prices and selling. No real research, no real plan. We just had to start clearing the junk out of the yard before my marriage fell apart. The hired help was not available after Wednesday, and I noticed that by Thursday afternoon, I had over $1,000 cash and I needed to not be alone, selling, with an infant. So, I went by my church and asked a retired friend, Craig, to come sit with me. He and a friend, Holly (a fellow stay-at-home mom), came to my rescue and helped us make deals and move junk. My husband made up some excuse about working out of town and left for the weekend. The truth was that he was totally furious about the circus I had created.

Nonetheless, by Sunday afternoon, we had cleared out most of the junk and given away the rest. I made over $7,000 after paying for the units, the workers, and giving my friends good tips for helping. There were a few remnants around the yard, but for the most part, most of the junk was gone. Nobody could believe we cleared so much stuff in such a short span of time. We kept the things we thought would be of value in a separate location. I'm sure we missed a ton, but the truth is that we had kicked butt and still had more to sell. It was genius.

So, I kept buying and selling. The Lord always knew when we needed a little extra and when we could afford to skate by. I always had cash in my pocket, and we were better off than we had ever been, even though I had an infant with special needs and no job. The craziest thing was that even though I had no idea if or how we would be able to afford me being without a job, we were doing better than ever. This was all part of the plan. I began to learn that when you trust God, with no reservations, He provides. His plan is so much bigger and better than ours.

Some of the cool things I ended up selling were a church steeple, an airplane, and even some old double-sided enamel signage.

The stories accompanying these finds are hilarious and will make a good read, so I'll work on that. But this is where I begin to transition into the reason I wrote this book.

I was at what I believed to be rock bottom. We were completely broke- physically, emotionally, mentally, and financially. When I quit my job, we had no savings. We had no back-up plans. What we had, though, was Jesus. The day that I turned in my resignation, I cried and cried. I took my oldest two kids out of the school we loved and put them into our neighborhood school. It was "Curriculum Night" and I cried through the whole presentation. I had no idea what I had done, and my husband was sure that I was overreacting. The truth was I knew I could not go on letting others care for my son. Taylin Cameron Bernard deserved to have his mother care for him. I will never regret pausing my life for three years. I was able to focus on him and only him during that time. Sure, I sold junk and started a business with very little capital, but it worked. The Lord showed up BIG time and took care of us.

When I say that the Lord showed up, let me tell you about some other things that happened when we surrendered to His will. We had no money. Since I was home, I was able to bargain shop. I created a grocery co-op with about 5 other families, and we bought fresh food in bulk. We were able to purchase restaurant quality food at a fraction of the price. I was able to keep our family grocery costs under $75 per week and we were eating like royalty. I also had time to look for additional help. I applied for the forgiveness programs at each of the hospitals we owed money to, and one by one, our debts were forgiven. One by one, day by day, things began to settle into our new normal. We had therapy almost every day in our home. I learned to do things we had never done before. I learned to tap into resources available that I didn't even know existed. It was a time of humility and humble acceptance of what we were dealt. It was also a time to be still and know that He is God. Because Yes!

# CHAPTER EIGHT

## CATASTROPHIC WHIRLWINDS

Three years is the magic number. Early Childhood Intervention ends when the child turns four years old. So, it was time to begin thinking about what was next. We had Taylin evaluated through the school system because kids with special needs can qualify for free services through the school system in Texas. We were doing well, and our needs were being met, but we still didn't have an influx of cash or capital to depend on. Taylin was doing well and meeting his therapy goals, so he did not qualify for special services through the school system. This was both a blessing and a curse. Taylin was behind in cognitive functioning and fine motor skills, but he was just that- behind. This required more personal time and specific, tailored interventions from me, but that was okay!

I had been praying about our next steps when one night, after being out all day junkin', our youth pastor called and asked if I wanted to go back to work. I knew school had already started for teachers and had already decided that as soon as the kids started classes, it was time to find a job. However, there were still open teaching positions that needed to be filled. I believe it was God's way of saving me from all of the "new teacher" in-service that I despise. I agreed to interview the next day and was offered a job on the spot. Like everything else, I had not mentioned that I had interviewed for a teaching position with Jason yet. I told the principal that I would have to 1- pray, 2- talk to

Jason, and 3- secure childcare for Taylin. Everything worked out, and by noon I was setting up a new classroom.

I landed a position at a terrific elementary where I quickly gained respect as an educator. As I write this, I am currently still employed there, and I can honestly say that the Lord has been good to us. The people I work with are outstanding, and the families I have had the privilege of serving have been second to none. They have taken my kids under their wings and loved them as their own.

All three of my kids had random things come up health-wise, but life happens. After a year of being back to teaching in a regular classroom, I grew restless. I can teach in my sleep. I remember praying for an idea of what could be next. That afternoon, we received an email about the University of Phoenix's doctoral program. It seemed like a long shot, but I applied and was accepted. Suddenly, I was enrolled as a doctoral student and flying off to Phoenix for my first residency. It was an exciting time full of possibilities and intrigue. At least, for me, it was a time to focus on the future and dive deeper into research. I became obsessed with Metacognitive Pedagogy (or the lack thereof, to be exact).

That year, Holly blew out her knee and had to have a total reconstructive knee surgery just before entering high school. She displayed a tremendous amount of resiliency, though, and even though she couldn't tumble, she spirited in on crutches and tried out for cheerleader while on a stool. It was the sweetest, most heart-wrenching thing to watch. But she did it. She was determined to continue to cheer, and her teammates voted her "Captain" for the leadership she displayed. After months of rehab, she was back at it!

Another thing that happened was Taylin entered kindergarten on the campus where I was teaching. I remember the "Meet the Teacher" night. We walked into the classroom, and it suddenly hit me… LETTERS. With all the physical obstacles in our way, I had forgotten entirely about letters, numbers, colors, and shapes. When the girls entered school, they knew all of that. I had not given one iota of thought to anything academic with my son- and I was a teacher. A doctoral student in educational leadership and I totally ignored academics because we were so focused on the basics like toilet training and pincer grips. It was most unfortunate for Taylin- and for us because we were facing yet another obstacle. Thankfully, the school personnel swallowed up our inadequacies and worked to catch

Taylin up to grade-level work. He struggles but is embraced by everyone and has no option but to succeed. This continues to be true as I write this.

What happened next is almost too difficult to discuss. However, it is the beginning of our next stage in the testimony that shapes this book into existence. This is where my life took a huge turn, and the worlds of modern medicine and research meet with trusting God's plan and relying on holistic measures comes colliding into catastrophic whirlwinds of exponential existence.

For months, Holly had been telling us that her back was hurting and sore. One night she left the football field crying after cheering. The next day, we went to an urgent care center because she was so sore and miserable. An MRI revealed a bulging disc, and my sixteen-year-old daughter was ordered to take it easy for six weeks. We were in the middle of football season during her junior year. No tumbling. No jumping. She could still cheer- just not kick, lift, or flip. Fine. Three weeks later, she was going to volunteer for our school's Fall Festival. Dressed in her cheer uniform, ready to do whatever, she bent down to tie her shoe and did not get up. She was in agony. At first, it didn't seem real. I was irritated that she didn't make it to my school but later realized she was hurting. I got home and iced down her back. The next day, we kept icing and moved up her orthopedic appointment to Monday. Another MRI indicated she had herniated her entire lumbar region (3 discs were herniated, and two were bulging). She was in so much pain. Nobody seemed to be able to help her, and she was crying out like nothing I had ever seen. It was horrible.

At that point, we began looking for a second opinion. We found a doctor who would actually listen, and he immediately hospitalized her for pain management. I cannot explain what all happened next because it seems so unreal. I just know that the following morning, she had a spinal injection that went terribly wrong. We ended up being transferred to a neurosurgery facility for the next nine days. The doctors called Jason and me in for a meeting around day seven and told us that Holly was going to require intensive therapy and care. They asked us if we needed help finding a facility for our daughter. Um, a facility for our 16-year-old daughter? Um, No. I AM the facility. Under no circumstance was I about to allow someone else to care for my daughter- no matter what it took, she would absolutely not be taken to a nursing home or rehab facility. We would do what we had to do to make sure that we did not allow this- not on my watch.

This is where the story begins to shift. I have consistently fought for my kids with passion. I have learned to navigate foreign worlds of medicine, doctors, insurance, public assistance, therapy, etc. I was about to embark on a journey unbeknownst to me, though. This was different. Holly's back injury was the springboard to learning to deal with things inside as well as outside. Because YES!

# CHAPTER NINE

## I'M THE BOSS

This chapter begins with a blog post that I created in December 2019, almost two months after my daughter's hospitalization, that subsequently landed her at home for three months. I am using my own words from the past in order to capture the emotions associated with learning to take control of my own destiny.

12/8/2019- I'm the Boss

A few weeks ago, my daughter hurt her back. This story will be in another post, but just follow along; you'll get the idea. She hurt her back, and we did everything the doctors told us- with fidelity. I tried so hard to make sure she had friends involved, stayed up with schoolwork, and even timed her medicine around family time. I mean, darn near killed myself accommodating the directives from the medical professionals.

Where did that get us? Nowhere. Things got worse. In fact, up until seven days ago, she had been told to try complete bed rest. This was a horrible decision, but we went along with the recommendation because it was from the doctors. Two weeks of bed rest. For my 16-year-old. Athlete. Cheerleader. Social Butterfly. Two weeks. The first week was somewhat okay, but then blood began to pool in her legs/ hips from laying around and taking too much ibuprofen- well, still within the daily limits, but too much for her body for too long- which is what we were supposed to be doing instead of using Hydrocodone. Next came the uncontrolled pain and ER visits to get relief. Again, muscle atrophy mixed with anxiety over the pain was leading to more pain, and seven weeks of nerve blockers, muscle relaxers, and opioids had left the medicine virtually useless to match the type of pain my daughter was experiencing. The moment I started getting really angry (there were several) was when the doctor at the ER asked, "Have you tried using a heating pad?"

NO KIDDING. Weeks and weeks of pain. Heating pad, ice, essential oils, CBD oil, massage, physical therapy, spinal injections, pain management, hospitalization, steroids, opioids, nerve block, muscle relaxers, walkers, wheelchairs, bedrest, meditation, cognitive training (psychotherapy), distraction…. you name it, we tried it. I was so mad. But he wasn't her doctor and really didn't know her story- he was just making rounds over Thanksgiving weekend. Fine.

What happened next is almost unbelievable. We had our follow-up appointment at Scottish Rite Hospital. Clearly, in the instructions from 2 weeks ago, it was stated that unless there was improvement through giving her body two full weeks of bed rest, she would be scheduled for surgery. We went into the appointment fully expecting to be scheduled for surgery. Instead, the Chief of Staff (her doctor) came in and explained that they really didn't think she would benefit from surgery- but rather an intensive inpatient therapy/ rehab program that uses a multi-disciplinary approach to pain management. A facility. What? Say that again. They said it again.

Fine. We talked and cried and cussed God for a little while. We prayed. We sought clarity and, as a family, stayed up all night weighing the pros and cons. We were told that the next day, Tuesday, we would receive a call with admitting instructions from our local children's hospital. So, Tuesday morning, I called to accept our sentence. The family services coordinator said that they had sent the referral for inpatient services and to be patient. So, I went to the grocery store to stock up on food for when we were gone, did all the laundry, and laid out clothes, notes, and instructions for Dad concerning field trips, club meetings, and after-school activities for the other kids. No call.

I started to feel like I was out of control. Then I remembered, "I'm the boss." I only heard that voice quietly whispering, but it was there. Instead of waiting around for the call, I insisted on going to lunch. Screw the doctors; let's just go to lunch. Take your pain medicines, and let's get out of the house. Done. At lunch, I remembered a crazy, loony, weird thing a friend posted about a foot detox. So, I looked it up. I'm the boss. I can try something while we wait. After the foot detox, we stopped and bought some equally crazy special filtered water that supposedly had healing power. Great. I'm the boss. I CAN do something.

By 3:30 that day, I spoke to the admitting hospital's coordinator for the pain management clinic. She assured me that they had received the paperwork, but that they were not scheduling new patients until February or March. WHAT? MIC DROP. You mean, my daughter is not being admitted today? She'll have to wait three months to get help? OH HECK NO. I couldn't believe my ears.

We hung up, and I sat there. I went and took a bath. Then, I called her doctor and left an insane message about how they promised to help, and now it was going to be months before she'd get help. I cannot even explain the type of out-of-body experience I was having. I looked for other places. I was clearly irrational, but I could hear "I'm the boss" in the back of my head.

Wednesday morning, my daughter already had a myofascial massage scheduled. Great. I was still pouring over how to help her, and my sweet friend, Kim, was helping me research other places and ideas on how to help. We looked at the pain management program and the "multi-disciplinary" approach. Okay. So, if we aren't going inpatient, what CAN we do outpatient? I'm smart. I'm capable. I can design a program for my daughter- right? I'm the boss.

While Holly was getting the massage, my phone rang. It was Scottish Rite. They said that they had no luck speeding things along, but really their job was to send the referral, and then it's up to the parent to be the advocate. Duly noted. I'm the boss.

After Holly's massage, we went to the children's hospital. I sat in the waiting room until I was able to speak personally to the scheduler, office manager, and subsequently the pain management nurse. She saw Holly. She saw me. She promised to try and get us an appointment earlier and would call if there was a cancellation. She also described the program and how things would go. They were completely different than what her doctor described, not necessarily bad- just different. So, we left a little hopeful, but no better than we went. When we got to the parking lot, I told my daughter out loud, "From this moment, I'm the boss. You're the boss. We are bosses. Nobody can tell us that we are on their terms anymore. We're going to have to do this together. Me and you. We're the bosses."

On the way home, my daughter got her first round of acupuncture. The next day, we went to the Spa Castle using a Groupon. We spent significant time in the healing saunas and whirlpools. We ate a healthy lunch and utilized the napping room. We rested. I kept my phone turned off for nearly 5 hours. On the way home, I noticed there was a voicemail. Guess who? The hospital. They were able to secure my daughter an appointment for Monday afternoon. Good. Being the ornery mom, I said to myself, "Good. I'll decide whether to show up or not because I'm the boss." Of course, we'll show up. We'll listen to their ideas. We'll decide if that is what we want to do. Monday.

Meanwhile, I had Friday to think about. I had already secured a second acupuncture visit and decided that I should post an update on my Facebook page for the enormous amount of people who had called, texted, or messaged me for an update. I just couldn't talk about things for a few days- 1- because I didn't know what was next -2- because the reality was daunting -3- because Holly was still in pain with no hope of finding her way out... So, I posted the update, and a friend, Angie, recommended Cryotherapy. Cool. I called. It was cheap enough, and so we went there before acupuncture. We also stopped and got turmeric since so many people were saying that the herb helped. Cool. I'm the boss.

Now, we still have to get to Monday's appointment, and now we're heading into the weekend. I decided that Saturday would be more than lying around. The best medicine is to distract, and the thing best for your heart is to not think of yourself. So, I told everyone in my house to get up. Put on make-up. Dress cute. I declared the day to be fun. Lunch, buying toys, attending the "Toys for Tots" fundraiser put on by Turn Key, pictures with Santa, and a car show. So that's what we did. We were literally out of the house for about 3 hours, but it was a good 3 hours. I heard laughter. We felt sunshine. We took cute selfies with filters. Good. I'm the boss.

Today, my parents are coming over. Today's therapy is family time and schoolwork. We're going to have a huge breakfast and watch football later. We're going to work on schoolwork and open windows and maybe even wrap a few presents. Tomorrow is Monday, but I am the boss. I make the decisions concerning my daughter's care, health, and wellbeing. There is something therapeutic about taking your life back and declaring that you are the boss. When there seemed to be nothing we could do to help my daughter, I refused to believe it.

Moms- we are the boss. You may not be waiting for medical answers. You may be struggling with how to help your kid in school or how to discipline with love and logic. You may not feel like you are the boss, but you are. Give yourself permission to be the boss. It's time that we act like we are the ones in control- especially when things feel so out of control. You are the boss this holiday season. You decide how many gifts your kids get, how much sugar they eat, and how late they stay up. You are the boss. If they have too much sugar or are overscheduled or spoiled, handle it. You are the boss.

I don't know who needs to do this, but repeat after me... I am the boss. I am the boss. I am the boss. I am the boss. I am the boss. I am the boss. I am the boss. I am the boss. Say it again: I am the boss.

So, there it was. That was the day that will go down as the epitome of turning points. I made the decision to stop accepting what I was given and start looking for solutions. What really happened that spoke the loudest to me was the Monday meeting with the Pain Management doctor. Holly looked her straight in the face and said, "Do you think I'm crazy? Is this all in my head?" The doctor assured Holly that she did have a very serious injury and the reasons why neurosurgeons did not want to operate on 16-year-olds. She explained that, yes, pain is real. However, our perception of pain is indeed somewhat in our heads. She began to explain cognitive restructuring protocols and ways to retrain our neuropathways so that we can manage our pain. The doctor also talked to me about my behavior. Every doctor and nurse for the last two decades has asked about pain on a scale of 0-10. We know that if you are having pain, you need medicine- right? The number helps us decide what type of medicine and how much- right? I had become used to asking Holly, "What number is your pain?" Here's the deal, though. Every time I asked her about her pain, it reminded her that she was in pain. Thus, I was causing my daughter pain inadvertently. This was the first behavior that we had to fix- and it was mine to fix.

The doctor talked and talked about different approaches to pain management. There were several options, including biotherapy feedback, physical therapy, massages, acupuncture, etc… Great! We had already begun doing most of the things she was talking about, and together, we made a plan. It felt good. Really good, actually. The facility was indeed our home, and I became a bonafide case manager and care coordinator. Because YES!

# CHAPTER TEN

# AFRICAN FROG PEE

Holly had three herniated discs. L3 (2mm) L4 (3.5 mm) and L5/S1 (5mm), and L5/S1 were sitting on the nerve root. According to the MRI, L1 was bulging, and L2 was protruding. The surgeons claimed it wasn't "that bad" and that at her age, with enough rest and therapies, the discs could shrink and could potentially go back to normal. They could also bother her for the rest of her life- depending on how her body healed. While surgery could offer immediate relief, it was not a responsible choice. Since most surgeons do not want to operate on a 16-year-old athlete if not 100% necessary, pain management was our best option.

To recap, pain management had begun three months prior. Holly did physical therapy three times a week for six weeks and had her first spinal injection. At that time, she only had one herniated disc on L5/S1... On October 19th, less than a month after the original injury, she was set to volunteer at my school. Hair, make-up, cheer outfit on... bent over to pull on her shoe and heard/felt a "RIPPPP" in her back. That's when life changed for us. That was the week she spent six days in the hospital on a ton of IV medicines to try to control the pain. She got a second spinal injection, and that's what we believe screwed her up. She woke up in a pool of blood from the OR and ever since that injection, her sciatic nerve was angry. Bad. Disabling.

Let's start with frog pee. The amount of pain Holly had experienced nothing short of the gnashing of teeth described in Revelation concerning Hell. Crying. Out-of-body experiences. Drama? You bet. But not the typical, attention-seeking drama- this was real. And heartbreaking. And scary. We were desperate. Besides calling out to the Father, face down in humble reverence, begging for mercy, we were lost. We began considering all options outside of modern medicine.

Jason knows a guy who can perform ceremonies where they burn African Frog Pee into your skin. You can only get these frog's pee from the jungles of Africa. They have tried to bring the frogs to America, but it doesn't work. Something about the African ecosystem makes these frog's pee do their thing. It apparently makes you swell up like crazy, meet God and then puke up all impurities in your body, leaving you healed. There are other ceremonies that involve putting acid under your tongue. I had spoken to his wife about scheduling him to come out. If African Frog Pee could help our daughter, well, it just wasn't off the table. I couldn't find much research about these ceremonies, but there was something comforting about knowing we had options outside of surgery and IV pain medicine. I decided to press hold on the healing ceremonies but committed to trying other things.

There were medical marijuana options. Medical marijuana had just started to be legalized in some parts of the United States at this time. In fact, a friend had a similar back injury about a year prior to Holly's injury, so he had traveled to Colorado and brought back some gummies. I had actual, fully loaded marijuana gummies that I considered giving to my 16-year-old daughter. But Holly was always the kid who gets drug tested, so I was hesitant to do that in case she actually did get better and wanted to return to public education. We agreed to the CBD oil massage and even purchased some from the herbalist. In fact, we contacted a herbalist, and she made a personal concoction specific to Holly's injury. The CBD oil and a deep tissue massage provided some relief. I don't know if it was the CBD or the thought of the CBD, though. Either way, it was something.

Y'all. We were desperate. I mean, we were considering African Frog Pee and Marijuana- but the truth is that we know that He is the only truth. We knew that if there were to be any level of healing, it would be because God had mercy on us. So, while we were seeking out wisdom from all angles, we had recognized the need for Him above all. On the way to one of Holly's appointments, we stopped by the church to pray with our youth pastor before we went. We truly believed that God would heal Holly and that He had given the doctors wisdom. We also believe that He has created lots of things on Earth to help us help ourselves. So, yes, we began at the top. Our friends, family, and strangers had been interceding on our behalf as well. We also asked several people to come over and do a prayer walk in our home. Every inch of our home was prayed over. We asked God to rid the pain and the doubt and the fear from our home and to teach us to trust and obey His will for our future. This practice was weird and somewhat like an exorcism but knowing that we were doing something felt good.

Bathing yourself in scripture is good. His word never fails. My friend, MaryAnn, sent me a ton of scripture cards that are easy to flip through- like index cards- with verses that are helpful. (You can find my version of these cards, complete with scriptures that have meant something to me on my website for free). To this day, I keep the cards on my mantle. When I am searching for counsel, hope, and encouragement, I always turn to His word. In fact, even when I am not actively seeking answers, I find the word of God to be an anchor for all that is. Another friend, Cindy, brought a devotional and a one-page printout of lots of scripture that helped us from going into that rabbit hole. So, yes. Start there. Bathe yourself in scripture and prayer.

Back to frog pee and marijuana. No, we didn't go there, but we were close. My advice to anyone seeking refuge is to start with prayer and scripture reading. Decide that you are the boss, and then consider some of the things outside of modern medicine that may help. When I finally decided that I was the BOSS, I took matters into my own hands. We learned about lots of options for holistic measures and some options that were too farfetched for us to pursue. Here are some things we found helpful:

Heat packs: rice packs you put in the microwave are nice. We were gifted a heat pack with a certain legume and essential oil. When opened, it seemed like they were split peas, but I'm not exactly sure what they were. The point is that a good heat pack with essential oils warmed up can provide a nice bit of warmth at the point of your ailment.

Cryotherapy is amazing. Cryotherapy is an inexpensive therapy that takes the body below freezing temperatures and pulls all the blood into the internal organs, thus richly oxidizing them and redistributing blood as the body thaws. You take all your clothes off (except underwear) and get into a space-ship type mechanism. You wear gloves and socks to prevent frostbite. You stay in the machine for just a tiny amount of time while your body temperature drops dramatically. The place that we went to also had a NormaTec machine that uses air to compress and decompress the joints. So, you call this a "Freeze and Squeeze" treatment. This helped Holly tremendously. We did this almost every single day for about a month or two. It was awesome.

Acupuncture: Gosh, y'all… you can sure get into a situation in acupuncture. The first place we went was $290 for the first initial evaluation. I had to think about that. I went to this other place, but there were homeless people all around, and when the lady's shopping cart fell over into the parking place I was about to pull into, I decided that wasn't the place for us. There is a doctor, though, in a neighboring town. He was a board-certified chiropractor and acupuncturist. He was super friendly and made Holly feel comfortable. His sessions were $65, and we did two sessions a week for about a month. Holly hated them, but they seemed to help. I think it was more of the idea of needles rather than the actual needles, but she went along with it. He also had natural pain medicines.

As far as medicines go, here's a few alternative options. Corydalis is an herbal supplement that acts like Hydrocodone. I took it to see what it was like, and I just got silly. Holly took it instead of the Hydrocodone and said it worked great. I don't know. I just know she didn't take opioids once we found the Corydalis. The acupuncturist sold them OTC for $20 a bottle. Aleve is the generic of Naproxen and is a 12-hour release- take that instead of ibuprofen- it's easier on your liver and lasts longer. Aspercreme with Lidocaine is the way to go for topical treatment and pain relief in specific muscle pain. Turmeric is also doctor approved- but get the kind with black pepper in it because it aids in absorption.

Yoga is encouraged as part of physical therapy. We went to a few sessions, but we never really got into it. The Cryo place has a beer yoga, and since Jason and I were long overdue for date night, we considered it. I digress. Does Yoga work? I don't know. I do know that stretching and meditation are good for all of us. I can't say that we did this with fidelity, but it was an option.

The Spa Castle in Grapevine, Texas, was ah-maz-ing. There are nine or so saunas and indoor and outdoor water pools that are like giant therapeutic hot tubs. We loved the Himalayan Salt Room. The entire room is made of salt. We started there and stretched. Then, we found the most help with the charcoal sauna and the 24-karat gold room. The color therapy sauna and the ice room were pretty awesome, too. We then put on our swimsuits and went outside. There are hot tubs with all different sorts of jets in all different places. It's hard to explain, but there are over a dozen hot tubs, and the two big pools have 10 or so different types of stations. So, you just kind of rotate through them and get massages from all angles. There are also napping rooms. We utilized that after we had a yummy lunch at the Korean restaurant. Now, I will warn you: In the locker rooms, you have the option to bathe nude. There are ten different tubs in each gender-specific locker room. You choose. We took full advantage of the spa. When in Rome?

The foot detox is interesting. The first time we detoxed was in a massage/ medical spa. Then, my mom purchased an Ionic Foot Detox Machine so that we could detox at home. Supposedly this machine pulls the toxins out of your body through your feet. We've all detoxed. Meh. It looks interesting, and all of us had different results. It seems a little hoaxy to me, but I firmly believe that if it works for you and you like it, do it!

Bentonite Clay- an Indian clay- is awesome on rashes and poison ivy. I had forgotten about that, but my friend reminded me of it. I bought mine on Amazon for about $9. You mix it with Apple-Cider Vinegar and apply. You then let it do its thing and then wash it off. This helped Holly's rash from the steroids. Also, it is the only thing I have found that works to dry out poison ivy.

Kagen water... IDK about that. We switched over to it for Holly. We got free refills at the C3 place. Does it work? I don't know. They say it does. People are convinced. I'm sure it doesn't hurt.

Essential oils and salt rocks- I don't know. I have salt rocks that I keep beside where I sit in the living room. They are said to draw out impurities in the room. They look fabulous and I figure they don't hurt anything, so whatever. I keep the salt rock light on most of the time because it is on the same outlet as my reading lamp. Again, whatever. Essential oils are something I am more convinced of having healing powers. I have a beautiful friend who spent several hours educating me on the benefits of several different oils that can benefit mood, pain, thinking, etc. I used them with fidelity for months. I infused, rolled, added to our baths, etc… While I believe there are oils that really do permeate the skin and add value to our being, I am not skilled or knowledgeable to offer advice. I can point you to my consultant, though. She's fantastic, and I do believe there is power in knowledge and that God created natural options for us. Therefore, I do embrace and recommend adding essential oils to your healing process.

Massages- Myofascial massage therapy helped with the knots in Holly's back. The muscles tensed up like Charlie horses around the spine. That is where most of the pain was. Think about having a Charlie horse in your calf…. it hurts so bad… then put that pain all over your lower back and mix sciatica with it. Poor girl. The massages helped- even though we weren't able to go deep tissue for quite some time. When Holly was on bed rest, we had the massage therapist come into our home. But, the other massages had been prescribed, and insurance paid for them. In case you didn't know, your doctor can prescribe myofascial massages, and insurance will usually cover a certain number of them. I highly recommend you talk with your doctors if you think this may help.

Diet- no sugar and limit dairy. Drink at least 80 ounces of water. Go gluten-free when you can. Eat green leafy vegetables. The ladies at the Cryotherapy place almost convinced me to buy a juicer. Apparently, celery juice is the best for anti-inflammatory healing. I don't know about that. Sounds gross. Unless you're talking about adding it to a bloody Mary mix… but that was not really for Holly…

Sleep and meditation. There are several apps that you can get on your phone for meditation and sleep training. I was too tired to need help falling asleep, but Holly explored several of the options. They call this biofeedback therapy. Cook Children's Hospital in Fort Worth, Texas, gave us a handout of about a dozen options that they recommend. Some are "babyish" according to Holly- but it makes me think about teaching your kids to meditate and breathe. They recommended no naps for Holly (super bummer according to her) and to get nine hours of sleep every night. No TV or phones- the white light distracts the brain from rest.

The next part is counterintuitive. Don't talk about the pain. Don't ask how she's doing or about her pain level. It sounds weird but asking about the pain reminded her of the pain. That's been my challenge. I had to quit asking how she's feeling and learn to observe her behaviors to gauge her pain. But, honestly, it's been nice. It's not that I don't care, it's because I do.

Education. We got to go to a class on using the tens unit properly. A tens unit hooks to your muscles and provides an electrical charge directly where the muscle needs it. We had one, and we just slapped it on where it hurt. Yeah, that will work. However, there's a way to target different muscles/ muscle families. Go figure. There's also a way to get into and out of bed. There's a way to go upstairs and get into and out of cars. I think we should all learn this.

Counseling- I would be remiss if I did not acknowledge the impact of counseling on our family. Holly faced a traumatic injury to her back. All of my kids have had life-threatening/ altering illnesses and injuries, actually. The problem is that as a caregiver, I had previously ignored the trauma I had experienced as their mom. I began to realize that I was suffering greatly from my own Post Traumatic Stress Disorder (PTSD). I was grieving what I had perceived to lose. I began counseling shortly after Holly and I returned to school in the spring. I had several sessions where my only goal was to be able to talk about our ordeal without crying. I was crying all the time. I cried in the shower. I cried in the car. I cried in the bathroom at school. I cried myself to sleep most nights. I usually cried in silence and alone- even when I was surrounded by others. Counseling helped me to talk about my feelings and explore ways to breathe. In the last session I had, the counselor asked me, "What is holding you back?" I said, "Nothing." Her next words are etched on my soul. She said, "Then, why are you still sitting on my couch?" From then on, I decided that I was done crying. Don't get me wrong, PTSD never really goes totally away, but I recognize what it is, and I have learned ways to breathe, talk, and work through feelings of doubt and fear. I am equipped with tricks and strategies that I will share as we transition into the next phase of this book.

There are lots of things that you CAN do to help that are non-surgical and helpful. Do your research. Ask questions. Try things. I have talked to lots of people that have lots of ideas: Decompression, atlas orthogonal, PX9000, tapping, psychotherapy, 360 machines, etc… Make good decisions for yourself and your family. I'll be happy to talk to you. I'll be happy to share. Watching someone you love suffer is the worst. And, if you decide to try the African Frog Pee ceremony, there will be no judgment here. Because YES!

PART TWO: BECAUSE YES

# CHAPTER ELEVEN

## YES!

YES! has become my new normal. YES! is an outward proclamation of my inward desires to dream, challenge, explore, investigate, inspire, educate, wonder, and pursue whatever presents itself. I learned the power of YES! as I began to explore the notion that life has so much more to offer than simply handling things. Each day we are given 24 hours to do whatever we choose. Each of us is given the same 24 hours, and it is up to us how we spend our time. I was spending my time worrying, planning, and responding to the things happening around me. Not anymore. Now, I say YES! to more of what makes me happy- even if it has taken a while to remember what makes ME happy.

Do you remember the scene from the movie "Runaway Bride"? Ike (Richard Gere) calls Maggie (Julia Roberts) out for not knowing what type of eggs she likes. Maggie had always preferred the kind of eggs that her fiancé liked. I had somehow become a Maggie in every aspect of my life. I was doing things because I was supposed to or expected to do them. I was not doing something because you weren't supposed to or because someone might not approve, or because we couldn't afford it. The truth is that I was just accepting what was happening all around me. Sure, I was in graduate school, but each day was full of commitments and expectations, and I felt out of control. And then, one day, I simply said, "No."

I don't even remember what it was that I answered "No" to. It might have been stopping by the store, deciding not to call someone back, or taking out the trash. I may not remember the scenario, but I remember how it felt. The first time I said "No" to something, I realized that I was saying YES! to something else: Me. Learning to say YES! to things that bring you joy is just as much about learning to say "No" to other things. Basic human psychology teaches that to have fun in life, you should do things that bring YOU joy. I had forgotten what I enjoyed doing.

One problem we face as humans is that sometimes we feel as though we have no choice in what is happening. Our basic perception of our situation is known as the "locus of control." Think of this idea as though you have a hula-hoop around your body. Everything inside the hula-hoop is in your control. Everything outside of the hula-hoop is outside of your control. In my "in-person" workshops, I would have attendees take a stack of index cards and brainstorm things they are excited about, nervous about, worried about, etc… We sit Indian-style in the middle of a real-life hula hoop and sort through the index cards to determine if the situation is in our control or not. If a situation is not in our control, we discuss ways to let go, approaches to the situation, and ways to regain control over chaos.

This is one of the ways we began to deal with Holly's trauma. We learned that there were lots of things out of our control and that the only way to regain a sense of normalcy was to restore our perception of control. This is also a way to cognitively restructure our perceptions concerning our situations. Learning to regain control of our own thoughts and actions yields a resiliency to adversity. This is what YES! is all about. At first, I was not listening to the voice inside my head saying that I was the boss. I was reacting to the advice of the doctors and experts around me. I was doing what I knew to be good, right, and true, but there was no control over what I was doing. Once I accepted responsibility for my thoughts, emotions, ideas, and destiny, I began to think more clearly. I began to understand just how much power I had, despite how defeated I felt.

I also realized that to embrace YES! I had also to accept what had transpired before so that I could move forward. I remember when Taylin was first born and receiving the punishing blows of diagnosis after diagnosis. A family friend said, "You were chosen to be Taylin's mom! How wonderful!" I was so mad. I mean, how could God choose to give us a son and then tell us that he would never sit, stand, or walk? How could I be "chosen" to be a special needs mom? It took me years to understand that through adversity, we have learned to trust, obey, and honor God's will for our lives. We were chosen to walk through the fire as a test of our faith, and He has honored us by delivering us from what could have been. I don't know why our son defied the odds, but he did. I will forever honor that deliverance by recognizing and celebrating all that He has done.

That's where the "because" comes into play. YES! for me isn't about just one day deciding to live differently. There are lots of reasons why YES! has come to fruition. YES! does not mean to live in reckless abandon- taking unnecessary risks- but to live with intention and embrace adventure. YES! means that because we learned to live by faith and by the power of our testimony, we have been granted another day and another opportunity to see His full grace in our lives. YES! is about taking care of ourselves and exploring what God has to offer in abundance when we open our eyes. So, the following few chapters will focus on saying YES! to the things that bring YOU joy. Because YES!

# CHAPTER TWELVE

## YET

The power of YET was one of the first tools that I discovered as I began to shift into the realm of YES! living. I was first introduced to this idea when a friend of mine shared a story from Genesis 32- when Jacob was wrestling with God. The two of them wrestled all night, and Jacob said to God, "I will not let go until you bless me!" I have taken this to heart and have embraced the idea that these struggles will materialize into blessings- eventually. There are many times in the Bible when God received praise through adversity. I decided to begin living in the joy of His promises- even if they were not evident YET.

The first sign of promise was when our youth pastor's wife came up to me after a morning of worship. She said, "You always have a smile. I don't know how you smile even though you are going through so much." I told her that my joy comes from the Lord. I didn't tell her that I cried all the time- or that just that morning, I had sobbed uncontrollably in the shower. I said out loud that my joy was from the Lord. From that day, I have consistently said that statement- to the point that I finally believe it. Blessings are abundant even amidst the daily grind of disappointment, diagnosis, and despair. If we sit sedentarily and wait to be happy, we'll never be joyful. I wasn't glad to be experiencing pain; I just knew that if I didn't choose to be happy, I wouldn't be. So, I raised my hands and thanked God for that day. I thanked Him for what was coming. I told Him that I would not stop wrestling with Him until He blessed us.

The power of our thoughts and words also started to resonate with me. I realized that what I said out loud had worth. As I said things repeatedly, I started to believe them. "My joy is from the Lord" became my mantra until I believed it so much that I began living joyfully because YES! I started studying with full intentionality- not just for my doctorate work but for my own personal gain. My research concerning metacognitive pedagogy began bleeding over into the world of self-help and affirmations. I began to dig deeper and deeper into my research for my dissertation and for my life. I learned that there is power in your words and thoughts. You have the ability to own your destiny, however quirky that may sound. You may not have received your blessings-YET. You may not have abundance- YET. You may not have joy- YET. You may not have that relationship, job, house, car, etc… YET. But, your words and your actions towards your desires are propelling your destiny straight ahead. Your job is to begin to take ownership of your future by acting in the present as though these things can and do exist. Because YES!

# CHAPTER THIRTEEN

## TIME

Let's start with getting real. Continue reading this chapter if you are real about getting real with yourself and your goals for the future. Some people will say that the first step is to decide what you want. Visualize your best day ever. Decide how you want to be remembered when you're gone. Choose a word to focus on for the year. These are all good strategies, but I suggest a different approach: find your locus of control.

We had medical diagnosis after diagnosis. We had mounting bills, little money to play with, and no time to do anything. Life felt out of control. One of the first things I did after recognizing just how powerful my words were was to start finding ways to take control of my life. This may sound weird, but I started parking on the opposite side of the parking lot. I was fat. Years of stress eating and hospital snacks and sodas had taken their toll on my body. I was still not in a place where I could diet. I was not ready to mentally commit to dieting, but I knew that I needed more movement, and I knew that I could control where I parked. Every day I took a few more steps. Then, I started doing goofy things like taking my car across the street during my lunch break so that I could vacuum the seats and throw away the trash. Pretty soon, I was eating less and getting more exercise- on purpose and on accident. I didn't make this huge announcement to begin to lose weight, I just started to give myself permission to take back my life, one decision at a time. The craziest thing is that the more control I felt over my decisions, the better decisions I started to make. I began fasting- intermittent and one meal a day (OMAD). I slowly cut out carbs and started going for walks instead of grabbing a beer. Pretty soon, my clothes began to get looser, and I found myself losing weight. People began asking what I was doing, and my best response was "YES!" I began saying YES! to things I could control and NO! to things that were not healthy for me. There was no secret, no plan, no investments, no fancy shakes, no supplements, nothing. Just a girl taking control over what was right in front of her.

I was working on my doctorate degree, working full time as an elementary teacher and part time university professor, and being mom to three active kids. My life was full of practices, games, livestock, and all the things that accompany teenagers. People would ask me, "How do you do it?" The truth was that every single minute was scheduled and intentional. Remember the power of our words? My first word was "intentional." Thus, I began to live with intentionality. Not only with where I parked my car and what I ate, but with where I spent my time.

I began to view my time as money, investment capital, and real estate. You and I both have the same amount of time, but where we choose to spend our resources is up to us. Time is a leveling playing field. 24 hours per day. The same 24 hours a day that Michelangelo had when he painted the Sistine Chapel in Rome. You cannot buy time, but you can choose how to spend your 24 hours every single day.

Giving myself permission to view time as money and learning to spend wisely gave me back my locus of control over scheduling without reservation. I began by getting real and honest with myself. I created a time audit to help me "see" where I was spending my time. For three full days, I wrote down where I spent every bit of my time- to the minute. Then, I kept recording my expenditures for the remainder of the week in fifteen minute increments. For the rest of the month, I kept an hour-by-hour record of where I was spending my time. I realized that I was making improvements in my spending even as I was collecting data.

If I spent my time on stupid stuff, then that's what I did. If I watched TV at night to decompress and got nothing else done, then that's what I did. I decided that if I allow myself the opportunity to watch TV, I could at least do sit ups, fold laundry, or clean the kitchen at the same time. I can still watch my shows, but I commit to take control over what I can control. It's okay. I sometimes still say YES! to just sitting still and watching my shows, but I am more conscious of what I allow myself to do.

Early mornings are the best "brain" time for me. I have excellent neuro connectivity first thing in the morning. My mind is fresh and ready to think. I can get more done between 3:00 a.m.-7:00 a.m. than I can for the rest of the day. Since I know that, I can plan to use my best brain power to tackle the things that take the most thought. For instance, I can write a paper in about an hour during the 3:00 a.m.-7:00 a.m. timespan. That same paper will take two-three hours to write after 5:00 p.m. My mind just does not work as well in late afternoon. I tire more easily and there are many distractions in my home after 5:00 p.m. To preserve time, I am cognizant of my natural body rhythm and the times where I am at my best. I capitalize on those times so that I can use the least amount of time to make significant progress. Likewise, I use the evening hours for mundane activities and household chores. By working through a specific, structured time audit, I am able to evaluate where I spend my time and how to make better investments.

I have learned to make adjustments in everyday tasks to improve my efficiency. I make a weekly grocery list that hangs on the fridge. My family is responsible for putting items they want and need on the list. Once a week, I have groceries delivered. While the initial cost of grocery delivery is higher than in-person shopping, I find that I only order what I need, and am committed to making a meal plan. Having meals planned saves my time. It also saves me money because I do not "hungry buy." Instead, I begin with the week laid out on the page and I write the weekly commitments next to each date. I plan easy and fast meals for the busy days. If we have a night off, I try to incorporate things that take a little more time to fix. I stick to somewhat of a schedule of Mondays-pasta, Tuesdays-chicken, Wednesdays-crock pot or grill, Thursdays-left overs or "fend for yourself," and Fridays- pizza- or go out to eat. The weekend meals depend on our kids' activities, but we like to smoke meats, grill out, or spend time creating meals together. I try to ensure that Sunday dinners are big and robust, like a traditional family meal at Grandma's house. My husband and I make our lunch for the next day before we even eat- that way we have our lunches packed and nobody steals all the asparagus before we get a helping to compliment the next day's lunch.

I keep novel and kid friendly food in our pantry or freezer for nights that I decide that cooking is too much. I keep things like macaroni and cheese, corn dogs, ravioli, and hot pockets on hand. I also keep ingredients to craft easy meals like red beans and rice, angel hair pasta, and scalloped potatoes in the pantry. There are rolls of turkey meat, sausage links, and a bag of chicken breasts in my freezer for times I need to piecemeal a quick dinner. My daughters know how to make those easy meals, too! They can fix dinner together when I do whatever else needs to be done, like times when I need a quick meal. If nothing else, they can cook together while I do whatever it is that needs done, like making a tutu for a Halloween costume, putting together science posters, or making a 100th Day of School project. Those are also the meals for the times when life spins out of control- like unexpected ER visits, hospitalizations, or accidents. While I try to control and plan for all things, I recognize that somethings are just not within my control. But I have a plan for that! Because YES!

Time is the most important part of YES! Understanding and accepting a generalized locus of control allows us to take intentional action for our future. Our time is ours to do with what we choose. To help me conceptualize investments, I also view time as investment capital and real estate. Unlike real estate though, you cannot produce more than you have. If you only have a certain amount of real estate, you cannot invent new properties. Instead, you can buy, sell, borrow, and cheat other parts of your portfolio- but that has a price. I mean, you can choose to eat unhealthily and buy bigger clothes, that is an option. Parking far away from the door, walking a few more steps, and choosing to drink water over soda or beer is another option within your locus of control. Your real estate options might be limited, but you get to choose where you invest. By choosing to plan and sticking with the plan for dinners throughout the week, I am choosing to not shop nightly and waste time trying to figure out what is for dinner. By choosing to have groceries delivered, I am investing in time to create healthy menus for my family with intentionality and respect for what we have planned as a family. By saying NO! to three-hour grocery escapades and haphazard purchasing, I actually am saying YES! to respecting and saving my time and money. If my kids want something, they put it on the list, and I try very hard to buy what they ask for if: 1- we have the money; 2- we don't have an abundance of food in the pantry; 3- they actually ate it the last time I bought it for them. I'm able to say YES! because I'm no longer making purchases with the hopes that my kids might like something new.

Now that we've talked about accepting our ability to control things in our lives, let's also talk about what we say YES! to. This was hard for me to learn. I love saying YES! to things, but I have learned that for every action, there is an equal and opposite reaction. If I say YES! to something, then I must follow through with it. This can interrupt my flow and requires me to say NO! to something else. One of the hardest things I had to do was to give up the work I was doing at our church. When I made the decision to go back to work, after being home for four years with Taylin, I could not keep the schedule I was living. I taught elementary school all week and then obligated myself to teach Sunday School. The latter obligation included having a lesson prepared, snack, craft, and open arms to embrace and invest in my students. By Sunday, I was drained. I had to let it go. I love Jesus and I loved teaching Sunday School, but I was finding myself resentful. I am so thankful I stepped down from that position, even though I still feel a little guilty about it. I think it is because I want to serve the Lord, but in doing so, I was sacrificing my family and finding resentment in my worship time. I am much better now that I have recommitted to praying with intention, worship, and conviction. There will be another time and way for me to serve, but that will be a different season.

Speaking of seasons, the concept of our season is so important to understand. This is where the power of YET comes into play. I read the sweetest, most desperate post from a new mommy of a precious baby girl and toddler boy. Bless her heart. She was exhausted beyond exhausted. The kids were up all night, one was sick, and her husband had just left for work. She was not griping; she simply had a hashtag #momming. I get it. I was there. It is important for you to remember that you are in a season. Give yourself permission to dream, wonder, ponder, and imagine what comes next. Yes, we must be aware of the present and accept our positionality, but we also need to recognize what season we are in. I have been in the Baby Season. I have been in the Stay-At-Home Mom Season. I have been in the Student Season. I've been the youngest mom on the team and the oldest. I get it. If you find yourself in an especially difficult season, remember that seasons change. Don't be afraid to ask for help and let others help when they offer.

Let's also talk about others. If time is like real-estate, we need to talk about our metaphoric neighborhoods. Does everyone tend to their own home? Do you help each other? Can you go to your hypothetical neighbor for an imaginary cup of sugar? How about $1,000? Would you lend your hypothetical neighbor your new lawn mower? If not, maybe it's time to think about who is in your neighborhood. I encourage you to enlist your neighborhood watch group; do an audit of your friendships and relationships. Sometimes people move into our neighborhood and cause a ruckus. We spend our time trying to make good investments and organizing our portfolio so that we can live in our own sanctuary. What happens, though, if we begin inviting others into our neighborhood? Your time is important. Investing in property that should be demolished is not wise in business or in your personal life. Sometimes it is hard to let it go- especially if there are memories attached to that old house, but it is the responsible decision. Ultimately, it will improve the value of the rest of the properties. Choosing to say NO! to the relationships that do not add value to your life is like saying YES! to those that do. Give yourself permission and time to manicure your own home, and really consider who you would want to cruise around the neighborhood in a golf cart full of enjoyment. Don't be afraid to gently evict those who aren't paying rent. If you keep investing and getting nothing back in return, it's time to cut your losses. They may have served as prime real estate at one time, but the market changes- and everything has a season. Some houses are meant to stay- because the bones are good. Treasure those. Take care of those. Let the rest go. Because YES!

Your time is valuable to your success with YES! (or any other goal setting, self-help, manifesting, life-coaching program). This is where it is essential to find out what IS taking your time. Be real. Where are you spending your time? Like a budget, this only works if you are real and honest with yourself. If you were planning a budget, but you forget your daily Starbucks, then you've missed a key part of saving. A daily $6 coffee equals $2,190 a year. It happens faster than you think. So does wasting time. If you want more time, start with being honest and looking at ways to "buy" more time. I have a 24-hour time document that I offer free of charge on my website. You can access it if you like premade downloadable documents. Otherwise, do like I do and use a lined piece of paper, labeling each line 12 a.m. through 12 p.m. Write down how you spend your time for a minimum of three days. I suggest doing this for a week to get a comprehensive idea of where your time is spent, but if you're like me, you can probably only commit to three good days of data. That's fine. We'll start there.

After completing the task, ask yourself: Where do I spend my time? Is this a good use of my time? What do I have to keep? Where can I trim? What can I combine? Can I use my daily commute to incorporate more worship/ prayer? Can I use my phone (hands free) to make calls that you know you'll be on hold forever for (doctors, insurance, bills, etc...)? Can I get up 30 minutes earlier? Can I go to bed 30 minutes earlier? Can I have groceries delivered and use those 3 hours to clean toilets and fold laundry? What CAN I do?

Next, start thinking ahead. Do you want to vacation? When? Can you take care of business before you go? Can you volunteer to help your neighbors today so that next week they will feed your dogs? As you are thinking and making more time for things that you enjoy, start making lists of the things you enjoy. Let's say you get an extra hour a week. That's four hours a month. What do you love doing? Can you build time into your month for four hours of fun? If so, you'll have 48 hours of fun this upcoming year! YES! If not a whole hour of "banked" time, can you take 10 minutes every other day to do something you really enjoy? For instance, if you give yourself permission to take a 10-minute hot bath every other day, well then, you've given yourself 1,825 minutes -or over 30 hours- of pleasure each year. Just like your Starbucks money adds up, your self-care minutes also add up. Decide right now to think about what makes you happy and decide to do more of that. I promise, you have the time. We all do. Because YES!

# CHAPTER FOURTEEN

## FORGIVENESS AND GRATITUDE

When my son was born and began receiving diagnosis after diagnosis, a friend of ours called and offered to help. As usual, I couldn't think of anything for her -or anyone- to do. People ask, "What can we do for you?" or they'll say, "Let me know if y'all need anything." Here's the deal- we have never asked for help. I have a hard time asking for help, and most of the time, I have no idea what I need.

One day, a friend called and said something I will never forget. She said, "You are so lucky! God chose you to be Taylin's mom." I was so mad. Angry. Hurt. Resentful. She said it so nonchalantly, but her words were infuriating. I made up a reason to end the call but kept hearing her words over and over: God chose you. God chose you. You are lucky. God chose you. I thought, "What kind of God allows kids to suffer? What kind of God allows parents to suffer? What kind of God…." I tried and tried, but I couldn't get past the question of why a God that claims to love us would allow our son to give us a son to be born disabled. How can that be a God thing?

It has taken me years to understand and appreciate my friend's words. The good news is that I learned that God chose us to be Taylin's family. That journey toward gratitude began with forgiveness. Earlier in the book, I discussed finding joy in our suffering. I struggled so much in finding joy in suffering. I had to learn to find ways to trust and obey God's plan for my life and that began with forgiving myself. I had to forgive myself for taking matters into my own hands. I had to learn to forgive myself for being so consumed with worry and fear that I missed several blessings in the struggle. I had received a blessing. I prayed for a son for years and I had a great one. Taylin has dark hair and big brown eyes. He's the best snuggler I've ever met. He looks at me and my heart melts.

The very minute I began to celebrate what God had given me; my life began to change. I began to put on makeup and drag my butt to church. I didn't want to, but I forced my hands in the air and began to worship like I had never worshipped before. I no longer allowed myself to feel sorry for myself. I still get scared, but I am no longer a prisoner of anger toward God for choosing us to be Taylin's family. Instead, I am so proud of the honor God bestowed upon our family. We are smart enough, strong enough, and willing to do whatever it takes to help our son. We are resourceful and our community of friends, neighbors, colleagues, and family are right beside us.

Being thankful took a shift in my thinking. It began with forgiveness long ago. I recognize now that Jesus paid the price so that we could receive unconditional forgiveness- forgiveness that we do not deserve. This book is not intended to preach the Gospel, but I would be remiss if I did not mention that learning to forgive myself meant understanding what Jesus did for us on a spiritual level. Our sins were paid for in full, thus allowing us to receive the blessings of God. For that, I am thankful. As I began to shift my thinking about thankfulness, I began to understand grace and gratitude. Grace is a deep level of understanding that is beyond compassion and comprehension. Grace is an extension of love. I learned that we all deserve grace at some point, and we owe it to ourselves to accept and otter grace as often as possible. The word I want to discuss at length is gratitude.

Gratitude is the quality of being thankful, being ready to show appreciation for, and returning kindness. Being thankful for something means appreciating the value that something or someone has added. For me, gratitude is so much more than thankfulness or appreciation. Gratitude is humbly acknowledging that I have been given a gift that I could not have provided for myself. Gratitude is the art of becoming the one who is so dadgum thankful, that I cannot wait to return the favor. With gratitude, I am constantly looking for ways to pay it forward because I know I could never repay what has been done for me. This is where I am. Once I learned forgiveness and started to be thankful for everything -good and bad- I realized that I had reached a place of Gratitude. I started to change my narrative and embrace a new direction. Sure, life was (and is) sucky at times, but I am full of humble gratitude for the grace we have been given.

One of the first things we did as a family was to volunteer at the Ronald McDonald House. I usually hate my birthday. July 5th is a day that has cursed my family and I used to think that if we just didn't talk about or acknowledge my birthday, it would go away. I lived like that for years. Until, one day, I embraced a new way of thinking. Instead of hiding out on my birthday, I signed us up to provide lunch for the Ronald McDonald House in Fort Worth, Texas. I roped in my family and friends, and we raised enough money to buy all the food. There were plenty of people who wanted to help, so we just did it. For three years, I spent my birthday providing lunch for the families who had kids in the hospital. My daughters stayed home to babysit Taylin, and the rest of my family joined me in serving others. Instead of hiding in the suckiness of the day, I chose to stop feeling sorry for myself and start serving others- because of gratitude. My birthday became something I looked forward to instead of hating. Because YES!

In January 2021, my middle child was hospitalized with a migraine headache. Gosh dang it was cold in that room. I mean, C-O-L-D. I had taken her in to the ENT, but we ended up in the hospital. It was cool outside, but I just had Crocs on my feet. She ended up being admitted to the hospital and I almost froze to death. I remember thinking, "WHEN… (notice not IF)… WHEN we get out of here and things settle down, I'm going to start collecting socks for other moms who find themselves with freezing feet during a child's hospital stay!!" By December of 2021, we donated 608 pairs of socks for moms and dads to our local children's hospital. It was awesome! So many people donated and helped to collect socks. I am proud of the work we did, but mostly I am excited that 608 pairs of feet are not freezing, thus the people wearing the socks can take care of their sick kids.

A final thought about gratitude began in the waiting room of the prosthetics clinic when my son was about fitted for his ankle/foot braces. If you ever need to eat a piece of humble pie, sit in a prosthetic's clinic and just watch the people come in and out. The babies. The veterans. The kids. If that doesn't get you, then come with us to Spina Bifida clinic over at Scottish Rite. There is always something to be thankful for. Always. #BecauseYES!

# CHAPTER FIFTEEN

## THE WHATIF MONSTER

There is a children's book by Michelle Nelson-Schmidt called, "Jonathan James and the Whatif Monster." The story is about Jonathan wanting to try something new, but a "Whatif Monster" starts questioning everything in hopes of stopping Jonathan. Jonathan does things he is afraid of and then ends up enjoying what he did. Everyone has doubts at some time or another. I remember when I first read Nelson-Schmidt's book at a teacher's conference long ago. I bought the book and the stuffed animal monster that is portrayed in the book. I remember it so vividly because it spoke to my being. I never thought of the Whatif Monster as a real thing, but I realized more and more each day that there are monsters everywhere. The Whatif Monster is just one thing that tries to attack us.

These days, I make things less scary by thinking in terms of fairies. I mean, if Jonathan James could be attacked by a Whatif Monster, why can't I be sprinkled with Whatif Fairy Dust? My Whatif Fairy Dust is sparkly soft confetti that sprinkles down from rainbow skies with all the goodness of lollipops and gumdrops. Why not? Why not have a Whatif Fairy to rain down goodness and kindness and hopes and dreams? What if she sprinkles miracles all around me and my family? What if she unites people from all races, religions, beliefs, origins, and backgrounds? What if she aligns all things- the Earth, wind, fire, and ice? What if all things really do work for good? Wait.

What? What if everything that has happened is exactly what was supposed to happen? What if all those circumstances of the past have led to this exact moment of Eureka? What if the diagnoses and the prognoses and the trauma, drama, and heartache were all part of a bigger picture?

Wait.

I have realized that all the things we faced have led me to YES! That is why Because YES! is so very important to me. Living with purpose and living by design is my authentic version of realizing that everything is important. We must face adversity so that we can relate and understand and offer hope to others. If things didn't work out in the past, they weren't supposed to work out, and vice versa. Life begins when we stop living it through the lens of the Whatif Monster. That is not where we are supposed to hang out. That is not the life God has promised us. We will face trials and tribulations. The scriptures declare that we will be prosecuted as Christians. The Bible does not promise that we will have perfect lives, but our lives will be perfectly designed according to His will. Our narrative should be more like Paul's... we should count it all as joy. Even though it is hard to see when we are in the storms of life, there is still another season just around the horizon. We get to be the ones to tell our stories. We may not be able to choose our circumstances, but we control our attitudes, perceptions, and actions. We get to decide whether we have a fairy or a monster. Because YES!

# CHAPTER SIXTEEN

## LET IT GO

Part of healing is learning to let things go. During my time off work with Taylin, I watched a lot of TV at night. He was fussy at night, and, since I was up, I watched a million hours of American Pickers and Storage Wars. I also became very interested in people's stories. I watched a lot of rerun Oprah shows. One day I watched a documentary about Oprah where she talked about the power of our story. The gist of her message was everyone has a story. We have our version of the truth, and the world would be so much better if we just learned to trust one another. She also talked about our connection to clutter. Oprah and Marie Condo (Japanese decluttering guru) discussed why people have clutter: We are attached to our stuff. The stuff tells our stories without us having to tell the truth.

I'm not sure exactly when I started seeing this truth. During my time at home with Taylin, I became a junker. I bought and sold junk. Some people let go of their stuff, and others hold on to what they thought the junk represented. I met all sorts of people and learned so much about the value of things. I started to shift my thinking about money and treasures as I watched other people's stories unfold. Honestly, it started making me sad to see deep emotional attachments to tangible items. I began watching people and how they chose what to buy. Some people were buying things like I was- to repurpose and sell. Junk was an avenue for revenue. For that, I was happy to be the middleman. For others, junk became part of who they were.

I remember when a lady asked if she could make payments on a dresser I had. It was a solid wood dresser with pretty knobs, but I remember only asking $120.00 for it. She wanted to pay $20 a week for six weeks. That meant that I had to keep the dang dresser for six weeks while she paid for it a week at a time. I offered to discount the dresser to $100 but denied her the opportunity to make payments because a big dresser takes up too much room for other junk. I did not want to hold a dresser for six weeks, and I knew my husband would disapprove. I think about that lady often. I wonder about her story. Did she really need the dresser? Why couldn't she just pay the $100? For me, a hundred dollars was just that- a hundred dollars. But then, I began to wonder why I was being judgmental. Who am I to question someone's ability to pay $100 for a dresser? I also wondered if I should have just given it to her? But, I was also trying to make money to feed my family, and I wouldn't make any money if I just gave things away. I gave plenty away, but this time, I wouldn't even let someone make payments. So, for me, the dresser became a bit of an obsession that I still think about.

I sold all sorts of things when I was junking. I know I've already talked about being a junker/ picker, but it set the stage for this chapter. I realized our joy could not come from things. Things hold space. We have things around us, and they take up energy. If we have too much going on, our brains are cluttered and using energy to take in the things around us. I began decluttering with the Marie Kondo's advice. At first, it was hard. I had a difficult time letting things go. It felt counterintuitive to what I was doing by selling junk to others. I began feeling guilty for buying and selling junk people didn't need. Then again, I was in a business that enabled people to hold on to things. My decluttering efforts continued even though I wasn't making much of a dent in the amount of personal junk I had acquired. Finally, I realized that I had begun to shift. When I say shift, I mean I was shifting things from one area to the next. I would tidy up a room, but the next room became cluttered. This went on for years.

When I started losing weight, I started letting go of other things. The idea that you had to start a diet on Monday had plagued me my whole life. Why Monday? Why not a Tuesday? I am reminded of my friend Joyce's story about her pot roast. She always cuts a pot roast in half before cooking it in the crockpot. I asked her why she did that, and she said, "Because my mom did." She called her mom and asked her why she cut the roast in half, and her mom said, "Because it never fits right in my crockpot." So, all this time, Joyce (and consequently me) have been cutting our roasts in half for no good reason except that Joyce's mom had a small crockpot? That is crazy!

We're all guilty of cutting roasts in half or doing things because we don't know any better. I started breaking the mold and learning to let things go. I had been out of the junking business for about four years, but still had junk around the house, yard, and barn. I started to lose weight and let things go- physically and mentally- it was time to start letting go of clutter. One Tuesday, I told my family that a dumpster was being delivered on Sunday. I warned them that things that were not in their place would be thrown away. They laughed. I warned them again on Wednesday; they laughed. The warning was repeated on Thursday and Friday. On Friday night, though, I began to make a pile of junk in the yard. Saturday, I spent all day making a massive pile of more junk, and on Sunday, the dumpster arrived early in the morning. I filled that whole dumpster up with junk, clothes, furniture, and everything in between within a few hours. Since my family finally figured out that I was serious and began helping, I ordered a second dumpster. We kept the dumpster all week, and every single day, we were working together and throwing out tons of stuff. I didn't even look in some of the boxes I tossed. I'm sure there was "good" junk, but I didn't care. Guess what? We all let go of so much. We laughed. We cried. We argued. And we let go of things we had held on to for way too long.

Do you know what else we did? We found seven staple guns, eight levels, eleven rolls of duct tape, and weed eater line. Things that we had lost reappeared. We found things we didn't even know were lost. Do you know why? We had become so busy that we didn't have time to look for the things we needed, so we just bought new things. We realized that we were spending money on things we already had, but we got so caught up with life that we lost things. Only, we didn't really lose anything- we just misplaced what we had. We are still not super organized, and we joke about being losers since we still struggle with organization, but we are much more conscious of what we have. We don't just run to Lowe's or Home Depot because something we had is missing. We look for it and then make a noble attempt to return it to where we think it belongs. My husband, kids, and I are still a work in progress, but we are better.

I chronicled my great dumpster adventure on Facebook. I think that I should have been given some major discounts or referral stipends, though, because many of my friends ended up renting these dumpsters and clearing out their messes, too! One friend ended up filling three dumpster loads from her property. It was the craziest adventure. But guess what? Giving yourself permission to let go of things in the flesh allows your mind to be open to the space. We tend to confine our thoughts to what we know. By letting go of the physical things of this world, we can begin to allow ourselves to receive what the universe has to offer. We can be open to new ideas, new processes, and new ways to dream, think, and live. Letting go of the junk on the outside was more about cleansing my soul of the troubles I had held on to for so long. I thanked the things I put in the dumpster. The junk had served a purpose—even things I bought and didn't use served to illuminate my spending habits. I have no regrets, and I learned a lot. I encourage everyone to purge. Let things go on the outside and the inside. Rent a dumpster. Go BIG and let it go! Because YES!

# CHAPTER SEVENTEEN

## GET LOST

This chapter makes me smile so big because I love everything about getting lost! When you need a break or an adventure, and you're unsure where to start, I suggest that you GET LOST! I wish I could take credit for this idea, but my husband invented this little family game. In the middle of one of my many "feeling sorry for myself" moods, my husband said, "That's it. Pack a bag. We're getting lost." I didn't know what to pack, but we all packed a change of clothes, a toothbrush, and a swimsuit.

Jason packed a cooler with drinks and a few snacks, and we just got in the car and drove away. We turned the opposite way we usually leave our house and found the first back road. At the stop sign, my husband asked the kids, "Left, or right?" They took turns deciding which way we were going until we got hungry. Then, we pulled over and had a picnic. The place had an outdoor chapel area, and Jason pretended to give a sermon. It was hilarious. We laughed and laughed and wondered where we would end up. It didn't matter, really; we didn't care.

We got back in the car and found a dairy farm. We pulled over and watched the cows for a long time. Then, we let my nephew drive. We pulled over again when we saw a baby owl injured on the side of the road. That wasn't a good idea because the mama owl was not about to let us get close to her baby. We kept going until we eventually decided to find a place to stay the night. I grabbed my phone and did a Priceline search for "Hotel Near Me" and found one with a pool. We grabbed a bucket of chicken and settled in for the night. The kids swam, and Jason and I just enjoyed each other. The hotel also had a game room. The kids played for hours while Jason and I just sat and talked. It was perfect. After breakfast the following day, we headed home. It felt nice to be away with no agenda, no destination, no rules.

Since our first adventure, we have perfected the rules. Rule 1: One backpack per person- no more. You should bring at least one change of clothes, a toothbrush, and a swimsuit in the backpack. Rule 2: Cell phones go in the center console. You can only use the cell phone to take pictures or book a room when you get tired. No cheating. Rule 3: No GPS or major highways. The point is to look around at new things. See what you see. Observe. If you know where you're going, you can't get lost. Rule 4: Bring two bags of microwave popcorn.

We started vacationing like this, too. We have a general idea of where we want to end up, but we don't make too many plans. For example, two years ago, we knew we wanted to head West. My husband had never seen the Grand Canyon, so we decided to head in that direction. We knew we had about ten days, and we were driving. So, everyone packed a backpack (we knew we'd wash along the way) and jumped in the car. We had no reservations. No agenda. No timeline. No expectations. We just headed West. We drove all night, arriving at the Painted Desert by dawn. We had to wait for the Painted Desert Park to open because we hadn't accounted for the difference between Texas and Arizona time zones. We drove a little off the beaten path and found a village of Teepees and totem poles to pass the time. It was an adventure full of laughter and random buffalo pictures! By the time we got back to the Painted Desert, the sun was just above the horizon and sparkling over the mountains. It was majestic and perfect! We spent the morning there and then drove on toward the Grand Canyon. We realized that we were on Route 66 and saw a sign for Winslow, Arizona. We taught the kids the famous Eagles' song as we veered off the road to stand on a corner in Winslow, Arizona- it was such a fine sight to see!

After lunch in a little diner, we headed back toward the Grand Canyon. On the way, we saw a sign for Flintstone's Park. We pulled over and hung out with Dino and Bam! Bam! for a few hours before heading up to Flagstaff, Arizona. When we got to the Grand Canyon, a huge rainstorm came out of nowhere, and the air became super cold! The canyon was dreary, so we grabbed a hotel room and hung out there until the following day. It was wonderful. We spent the day hiking and exploring the Grand Canyon. Jason and Dani don't like heights, so they nonchalantly joined a random tour group that stayed around the rim while Holly, Taylin, and I went down the trails.

When we met back up, we decided to keep driving to Las Vegas. Why? Because YES! We spent a few days playing in Vegas at Circus Circus (they have a waterpark) and seeing the sights. Jason and I didn't gamble too much, so we just spent our money on new school clothes for the kids. We didn't intend to school shop for the kids, but there were a few stores on the strand near our hotel with amazing sales. It kind of just happened. When we got tired of Vegas, we decided to head back to Texas. On the way, we saw a sign for Tombstone, Arizona. I love the old movie by the same name, and the little town was super cute. We watched a gunfight and took a covered wagon tour. Finally, we headed home from a vacation that I could have never planned. Our "Get Lost" style of vacationing has taught us that it doesn't matter what we are doing or where we go. Being together is an adventure in and of itself. Because YES!

# CHAPTER EIGHTEEN

# MANIFESTATION

This chapter may be the strangest thing I have written. Learning to manifest what I want has been a struggle. I lived so many years in fear of what was next. I constantly thought about the next diagnosis, or the next hospital stay, or the next unexpected setback. I expected things to go wrong and not to be able to afford what I wanted- so much so-those bad things kept happening, and I stayed broke. Finally, I realized that what I was living and expecting was precisely what I was given. The Universe hears us. By saying I expected something to go wrong, it meant that something would go wrong- so I was right. By saying that I couldn't afford something, I limited what I could afford. Again, I was stuck in a cycle of stinkin' thinking.

My mom bought a book for me when Taylin was about four years old. She gave another copy to my sister and asked, "For Christmas, will you read this book with me?" We both agreed, but I don't think my sister ever actually read it. Mom and I did, though. The book was titled The Magic by Rhonda Byrne. In this book, Byrne discusses the idea that magic is realized through gratitude. For example, the more thankful you are for something, the more you receive it. The book lays out a 28-day process for the reader to do little things each day to express thankfulness. I halfway participated in this hokey pokey thing my mom wanted to do until I noticed a shift in my thinking. Not a big shift (because I wasn't all in), but a slight nudge. On one of the days, you were supposed to put a dollar on your bathroom mirror and thank it. I said to the Universe, "Thank you for the money I have. Thank you for the money I have had and thank you for the money I will have." This process was like the Marie Kondo method of thanking things for their service and then letting them go, except in this situation, we were holding on to the money and thanking the Universe for money we didn't already have. Great. Weird. You got it, Mom. I'll do it.

I also chose a rock, thanked it for helping me to remember to be thankful, and kept it beside my bed. I made a daily list of ten things I was grateful for. At first, I played along for my mom's sake and thought it wouldn't hurt to be a little more optimistic. After completing the book in 28 days, I felt a little better. But, as the old saying goes, "Energy flows where your attention goes," and I fell back into the everyday grind. My dollar was taped to my bathroom mirror, but I stopped telling it, "Thank you." Eventually, I forgot that it was even there except when I cleaned the bathroom mirror. I am revealing my handicap in recognizing the power of our thoughts. The Universe responded to my gratitude and began to reveal little bits of magic, but I was too deep in my pessimistic outlook to see it.

It took about a year before I realized that there might be something to all the talk about manifesting what we desire. As usual, I didn't just dabble the second go around with learning to manifest what I want. I went all in and began researching how to maximize my manifestation power. I'm still all in and am learning to allow myself to feel joy and gratitude for the experiences that have formed who I am. This entire book has been a way for me to chronicle the struggles and difficulties that have led me to this place. I hope that someone reading these pages will realize that I didn't just arrive at a place of YES! but that there have been serious struggles along the way. I have lived through death, despair, diagnoses, and illness. I've been so scared that I found it hard to take my next breath.

While our situation has been exponentially different than others, the truth is that we've all faced our own set of battles. You may not have had a son born with Spina Bifida or watched your perfectly healthy daughter suffer life-altering pain. You may have never wondered if you have enough change in your closet to buy another gallon of gas to get to the hospital. You may have never taken the toilet paper from your place of employment because you couldn't afford your own. You may have never skipped a meal so that you can feed your family. You may not have quit your job or applied for welfare. You may never have had home health pack your wounds or had to give your child CPR in the back of a minivan. I hope you never do. But, realizing that we all have a story is important. Even more important is realizing that we are the one who controls our narrative. Your story up until this point is in your past. You do not have to live the way you have been living if you make different choices. You are the author of the present, and the future is yours if you allow yourself to get out of your own way.

I was in my own way more than I realized. My negative vibes and expectations for defeat defined my story. I blamed my weight on being depressed or unable to pay for healthy foods. I blamed the doctors for not being able to help my kids. I blamed my husband for not making more money. I blamed God for not showing us favor. Whoa. I was out of control with my blame game. As I began making changes, I realized that I was the one responsible for what I put in my mouth. I was the one not asking God for what I wanted. I was the one who wasn't thankful for the money we did have, and I showed little regard for what we were given. It has been a process, but each little thing has led me to the place I am now, and I pray that you can learn from my years of doubt, fear, and the perception of lack of money, time, energy, and resources.

I am not saying that I have everything that I want. That would be a lie. But, the things that I genuinely desire have been given to me abundantly. I may not be rich (yet), but I have learned how to let things go that weigh me down and be grateful for what I have. Each new day brings about the same opportunity to give thanks. I have led book studies with like-minded people who have taught me many ways to embrace the affluent lifestyle that I desire. I started by rereading The Magic. If you've never read it, I would recommend doing so. "Make Your Bed: Little Things That Can Change Your Life" by Admiral William H. McRaven is terrific. Admiral McRaven talks about his time as a Navy Seal in that book. His story is extraordinary, and his message is simple: little lifestyle changes can change your life. By making your bed each morning, you set yourself up for success. Even if the day sucks, you can end each evening knowing that you at least did one thing right- you made your bed. I also read books like, You are a Badass: How to Stop Doubting Your Greatness and Start Living an Awesome Life by Jen Sincero, and The Subtle Art of Not Giving a

F\*\*k by Mark Manson. These books have cuss words. I had never read a book with cuss words (lots of them), but I liked the message and appreciated the raw commentary. I learned to embrace the language even if I giggled a little when listening to the audible versions.

Speaking of audible versions, I don't always have time to read. I like reading, but I don't always have time to sit down and read. So, I buy the audible versions of books. I like hearing the author read, too. It makes the book more personal to me. When I go on my walks, I like to listen to words of empowerment and story. I like hearing these when I am out walking because they give me the strength to go on. There's an old song that we used to sing in Sunday School: "Oh be careful little eyes what you see, oh be careful little eyes what you see... For the Father up above is looking down in love, Oh be careful little eyes what you see." The subsequent verses include little ears what you hear and little mouths what you say. I like that. It reminds me that we need to be careful what we listen to and what we say, in general. If all we hear is the World saying, "No" or "You Can't" or "Not Now," then that's what we begin to believe. We must be careful to choose what we hear and who has our ears. I recommended books with cuss words, but it isn't about the language; it's about the message. If we're only listening to the World's negativity, then that is what we hear.

Another book that I have found enlightening is Carol Tuttle's "Remembering Wholeness: A Handbook for Thriving in the 21st Century." Tuttle talks a lot about living with joy and letting go of lack, pain, and suffering in this book. I found her straightforward approach to ownership of our lives most enlightening. While participating in an online study of this book, I realized that we are in charge of our reactions, actions, and situation. I am the only one to blame if I live in pain, lack, and suffering. We allow ourselves to get so tied up in the NOW that we forget to define our reality. Our versions of Truth become skewed by what we believe to be true in the moment. We fail to look around and remember that we were designed to be a part of something bigger and more significant. Studying these books and hearing from others about overcoming difficult situations helped me to be a better version of myself.

Another method that helped me overcome negative self-talk was working with a life coach. My life coach, Jeanie King, is a friend of my mom's who had been following our story and wanted to help.

At the time, I was too broke to hire a life coach, but my mom asked me to speak with her. She had experienced a back injury similar to my daughter's and had written a book called Giddy Up. This book talked about getting back on the horse that had caused her so much pain. In life, the message is the same. We must embrace our situation and find ways to Giddy Up. What we tell ourselves is our story and our version of the Truth. Jeanie King has helped me realize the power our words and thoughts hold. What we put into the Universe is what is given back to us. If we put negative thoughts and emotions into the Universe, guess what? That is what we'll get in return. Dadgum. I don't need any more drama.

I have started visualizing and creating the life I love. The Universe has responded in more ways than I can explain. You can have anything you want in life. The choice is yours to embrace and give thanks for what you have been and will be given. But, on the other hand, you can also choose to wallow in your pain, lack, and suffering. The more attention you give to positive affirmations, though, the more energy you attract to bring those things into fruition. You don't have to do anything, but that's exactly what you'll get in return. Passionately embracing your desires makes those things more likely to come into existence. That is the rule (even if it took me a long time to figure out). I am not PollyAnna. Life still happens. Bad things still happen to good people. But I firmly believe that our response to events brings about the results we desire- even if the blessings are disguised. We may not know the answers or reasons why things happen. I don't understand why babies are born with Spina Bifida. I know that there are blessings all around us, and I wish that I hadn't taken so long to figure this out. Just like getting lost is more about being together, learning to trust is about learning to let the blessings reveal themselves. When we force something, we deny the ultimate design of God's blessings to flow around us. His plan is always better than anything we could have dreamt, so try to embrace what is happening and let things go. Get lost. Throw things away. Do what you must do to learn to embrace YES! Manifest your desires. Because YES!

# CHAPTER NINETEEN

## DO MORE YES THINGS

So, we've been through the hard stuff. We've been through the chapters about letting things go, getting lost, and manifesting what you want. Now, let's talk more about YES! It comes down to basic Human Psychology 101: To be happier in life, you should do more things that you enjoy. The people who appear to be enjoying life are the people who are doing things that they enjoy- right? The problem is that the older we get, the more we tend to forget what we enjoy doing. We get so busy doing what we must do that somewhere along the way, we have forgotten about doing things we enjoy doing. Of course, this does not release us from all responsibility. But, we have to make a conscious decision to incorporate more Joy into our lies intentionally.

One gorgeous, brisk, sunny spring day, two friends and I found ourselves free of obligations. We were sitting in my living room staring at the TV while the kids played when I said, "Let's go do something fun!" Everyone smiled and said, "YES!" and then proceeded to talk about what we should do. We had difficulty figuring out what to do without spending a ton of money. At that moment, I realized that we three grown women had lost ourselves in our own lives to the point that we didn't even know what we enjoyed doing. What was fun? Finally, I told everyone to get in the car because I had an idea. I love water, and there is a public lake with a park about 20 minutes from my house. So, we loaded up and started driving. I like tea, so we swung by Chicken Express and got a sweet tea for everyone. When we got to the lake, I grabbed the kites I had in my closet for years, and we attempted to fly kites down by the lake. That ended up being a dumb idea because it was much too windy to fly kites, but we were out in the sunshine, drinking tea by the lake, and playing with our kids. On the way home, I noticed a patch of bluebonnets on the side of the road, so we stopped and took ridiculous pictures in the bluebonnets (an authentic Texas tradition). The images were absurd because the kids were messy with mismatched clothes and messy wind-blown hair, and the bluebonnets were not ready for pretty Spring pictures. Nonetheless, we went. We played. We did something that we enjoyed- even though it was a struggle in the beginning.

When we returned, we talked about why it took us so long to figure out what we enjoyed. I am not sure we ever came to a consensus on the rationale behind our inability to determine things we enjoy. Still, we agreed that it was not okay. We made a pact to think of things we enjoy doing and to do more of those things. I took the lead: I like having dinner on the patio. I like going to the movies. I started naming a million things I like doing but… and there it was… the but…but it seems that everything costs so much money when you have three kids- or even when you don't. The challenge then became to make a list of things we enjoy doing but don't cost too much money.

Just like everything else in my life, I went all in. I started making lists of things I enjoy so that I could do them without reservation. I realized that there were so many things I enjoyed doing. That may sound weird to other people. The key is to do more things I enjoy doing, so what the heck. I enjoy fishing. I really do. I enjoy cooking. I enjoy going to the grocery store and picking out meats and vegetables. I enjoy cleaning and preparing food. I enjoy grilling, baking, cooking, and making dinner. I even enjoy doing the dishes - just not all of the time. I enjoy the smell of a clean house. I enjoy looking in a clean mirror. I enjoy taking hot baths. I enjoy drinking coffee in the hot tub. I enjoy fireworks. I enjoy blowing the porch off with the electric blower. I enjoy sitting outside. I enjoy a good fire- the kind that is so hot you can see blue flames at the bottom. I enjoy swimming and lying out by the pool. I enjoy drinking ice-cold water- right when the ice is almost melted, and the water is cold! I enjoy scrolling on Facebook. I enjoy taking long walks and having conversations with friends. I enjoy playing card games and watching football on TV. The list that I began to craft was not an elaborate Life List or Bucket List, but a definition of the things I enjoy the most. I realized that I do lots of things every day that I enjoy- I just wasn't taking the time to appreciate them. I do have time for things that I enjoy, but I have to realize what they are and appreciate them. The simplest things that we appreciate yield significant results when we express thanks. I think we can get so caught up in thinking about having to make time for things we enjoy that we forget to enjoy the little, everyday things. As a result, we overlook the Joy already present.

I have made a more noble effort to engage in things that I really, really enjoy that are not limited to the ordinary. For instance, I love live music. I know Friday nights are always a little tricky because we are usually exhausted from the week. Still, I have made a conscious effort to listen to live music and have dinner on an outdoor patio. It's not big, expensive, or elaborate, but it is dinner outside on a patio, listening to live music. I love that. I think it's important for my kids to see that I am placing importance on having fun in life, too. Yes, we may be tired, but we will have fun! I also stalk my friends and see what they are up to and where they go. If there is a restaurant or a venue that looks fun, we go. If I want to have a pinata and a taco bar to celebrate Cinco de Mayo- even though we have no cultural ties to the holiday-we do it! A friend of mine, Kasey, would always buy one of those cakes on the clearance racks at the local bakery. She would have the baker write on the cake, "Happy Unbirthday to ...." And then choose someone in the group to celebrate. She loves store-bought cake and there is always something to celebrate. I love that! Because YES!

What about the things we have to do that we do not enjoy? Well, you just told the Universe that you don't enjoy something, so you denied yourself the opportunity to enjoy it. That sounds weird. I do not enjoy a root canal, but if you need a root canal, you may as well find something to celebrate. Suppose you focus on the idea that we are fortunate to have dental care available and that our teeth are essential to our health. In that case, it is easier to find Joy in the circumstance. Be thankful you can afford dental care. Be grateful you have teeth. Be thankful someone can help you. Be thankful for medicine. Find something to be thankful for- even the things that do not bring you Joy. Being thankful for what you are experiencing allows the Universe to respond with Joy. I know I might even be rolling my own eyes a little, but it is just the Truth. I've never been thankful to have to put one of our dogs down, but I'm thankful for the Joy they brought to our lives. I'm never thankful to be sick, but I am thankful for medicine. I'm never thankful to watch a loved one suffer, but I'm thankful to have people I love. I get it. It is not always easy to find things we appreciate and enjoy when our situations feel bleak. However, we can control the narrative of our lives. We are the ones who must respond to situations, and if we live in a constant state of fear, lack, or suffering, then that is the choice we make. Choosing to look for things to be thankful for can be difficult, but the difference is exponential. You can decide to be angry. That is your choice. You can decide to be bitter. That is your choice. You can choose to forgive or to hold a grudge. That is your choice. Choosing Joy and choosing to say YES! leads to a more enjoyable life. I do not guarantee you will not face adversity or difficult situations. How you choose to view your situation, though, is really up to you. Because YES!

# 99 YESISMS

This section of the book will focus on YESisms that have evolved over a full 365 days of saying YES! These lessons are the very best of the YES! They encompass and celebrate the most basic to deep universal truths. Learning to say YES! has been a process for me. This process has helped me heal and grow. Now, I share these with you! Here is what I have learned through my intensive study and quest for understanding.

## 99 YESISMS

1. Our thoughts lead to words. Words lead to beliefs. Beliefs lead to habits. Habits form our reality.

    Who you are is who you are in the habit of being. From this moment forward, take ownership of the narrative of your life. When you begin to think differently, you begin to speak differently. Your words help craft your belief systems which mold your habits. Your habits form your reality by creating new neuropathways. You choose how you respond to situations. You choose how you internalize struggle. The easier it is to do something, the more we do it. Resistance prolongs change. So, practice thinking positively! Speak positively! Believe in goodness! Choose YES!

2. You are worthy of happiness.

    Because YES!

3. There is power in YET!

    American Psychologist, Carol Dweck gives a terrific Ted Talks about the power of YET. Instead of thinking about what you can't do, add the word "YET" to the end of your sentence. For instance, I can't afford a pedicure YET. I haven't climbed Mt. Everest YET. I haven't beat cancer YET. Whatever it is that you are struggling with, turn your thinking in a different direction by adding the word YET to the end of your thoughts. You'll be surprised how quickly your mind begins to shift and the Universe responds. Because YES!

4. "In order for our wildest dreams to come true, we must dream wildly." -Jeanie King, CEO of the Beautiful Network of Women (B-NOW)

> A dear friend of mine, Jeanie King, introduced me to this idea. She says that if we want our wildest dreams to come true, we must dream wildly. I began to dream wildly, and the Universe began to respond. Now, my dreams are so big that I sometimes pinch myself to see if I am alive or stuck in a purple world. The truth is that the bigger we dream, the more we allow ourselves to receive exponential blessings. Don't settle for little miracles. Go big! Because YES!

5. Wisdom's Wages and Folly's Pay by Howard Pyle is worth the read.

> In this short story, Simon Agricola pays for a piece of advice. The advice was, "Think well. Think well. Before you do what you're about to do, Think well." He then overhears a plot to kill the king and uses the advice to save the king's life. The point is that the advice rings true for all of us. We should always think before we speak. Think before you hit send. Think before you post on social media. Think about the consequences of your actions. Even more than that, think about the unintended consequences of your actions. Also, think about how inaction is also a choice. Whatever you are considering, just think well. Because YES!

6. Why not me?

> A few years ago, I heard a young volleyball player who had won a medal at the Olympics speak. I can't remember where I was, what year she played, or what the exact story was, but I remember her words, "Why not me?" loud and clear. She talked about being a small-town girl with big dreams. She talked about how the teammates made fun of her country accent and how nobody really paid much attention to her in high school. I could relate. I tried out for cheerleading four times in junior and high school. I never made the team, but I went on to be the cheer/dance captain for my

college. I also graduated valedictorian and have since finished my doctorate degree. Little ol' me from a little bitty town in the middle of nowhere. Why not me? Good things can and do happen to all sorts of people. Why not me? Because YES!

7.  Trust that each new day has new opportunities.

    I want to look in the mirror each morning and have the mirror think to itself, "Oh boy! She's up again!" I want my tennis shoes to ask, "Where are we going today?" I want to awaken before my alarm clock because I am so excited about whatever the day has in store for me, like a puppy who can't wait to play. The energy of the day is new and fresh. I do not want to waste one more day hesitating or dreading whatever is next. I get to choose how I approach all situations- even the difficult ones. On difficult days, I find that meditating and preparing for goodness, mercy, and grace helps. If you know you have to do something yucky, find a way to have fun in between. On our Spina Bifida clinic days, we go to Chuck E. Cheese. For surgery days, we get new funny socks. Plan to have a good day despite whatever it is you are up against. Because YES!

8.  "Instead of worrying about what you cannot control, shift your energy to what you can create." Roy T. Bennett, Author of "The Light in the Heart"

    I shared a bathroom at work with a friend of mine. She had this sign up in there with two little bluebirds that said, "Why pray when you can worry?" It made me laugh. There have been times when I didn't know how to pray. Worrying was easier. But I realized that worry steals joy- and if we are trying to increase our joy we should worry less. Nobody really talks about what to do if you aren't worrying, though. First, I recommend that you pray and cast your cares on Him. He cares about you. I also recommend that you shift your energy by recognizing what you can and cannot control. If something is out of your control, figure out what you can control and use that energy to create what you want. You are smart. You are capable. You are creative. You CAN do something. Stop making things difficult. Let go of things beyond your control and stop worrying. Pray. Create. Because YES!

9. Excuses are just that. Stop that.

Yep. Just stop. In his book, "Tacos and Chocolate," Drew Myres talks about stopping with the excuses. If you want to lose weight, look better, and feel better, do it. Exercise. Eat right. Talk to your doctor. Make a plan. Start today. Don't wait. If not, that's cool too. But, don't sit around complaining that you are overweight while lying on the couch eating Hot Cheetos and drinking Mountain Dew. There is no excuse for an excuse. Own it. If you mess up, own it. If you want to make a change, do it. Don't make an excuse, though. When the lights go out at night and you are alone, you can't hide from your own truth. Just stop. Stop lying to yourself. Stop lying to others. Just stop. Enough. (This is as much of a reminder for me as it is for anyone reading these words.) Own it. Because YES!

10. Start with something you CAN do.

One of the things I started doing when I decided to lose weight is to park in the farthest parking spot away from my classroom door. I knew I had an addiction to food, but I was at least in control over how many steps I got each day. I took control of one thing: where I parked. Regaining a sense of control helped me make better decisions in other areas of my life. I began eating better. I stopped drinking alcohol for months. After I learned to do one thing, I took control step by step. Start with something you CAN do. You may not be able to predict the outcome of your tests, but you CAN paint your nails. You may not be able to buy a new dishwasher, but you CAN buy a new dishtowel. Stop thinking you can't do something. Remember to add YET to the end of your sentences, stop making excuses, and start with something you CAN do. Because YES!

11. Do something your future self will thank you for.

Time is a thief. We look back and wonder where all our time has gone and why we haven't done more. If you are like me, you find that you have so much to do and so little time. This YESism can be a grand gesture of self-care, or it can be as simple as loading the dishwasher before you leave the house. Just this morning, I took a baggie of leftover chili from the freezer and put it in a crockpot. My old self would have thrown out the leftovers and not messed with freezing them for a future meal. Today, I was thankful I had a meal that was ready to go! This is just an example of doing something that you will be thankful for later. You can also establish routines that help you achieve your goals. For me, this looks like decluttering the living room so I can pick it up easier each evening. I like waking up to a clean space, so I make a point each night to put things back where they belong. In the morning, I am thankful for my efforts even though I don't think much about it anymore. Be nice to yourself and develop habits that help your future self. Because YES!

12. Give thanks for blessings that are on their way.

Learning to live in abundance is about recognizing that we already have what we need and that the only thing we really need is Jesus. Your blessings are already here on this planet. The energy, the desires, all of it. Whatever you want and need already exists. Your job is to be thankful for what you have and to attract more of what you want. To increase the flow, give thanks for the gifts that you have already been given. When you want more money, give thanks for the money you have and watch it multiply. When you want recognition, be thankful for the times when you have felt valued and recognize someone. Be thankful always and in all ways. Know that your next blessing reflects your gratitude for what you have been blessed with already. Because YES!

13. It doesn't take much fire to light up a room. Share your fire.

The great "Snow-vid" in 2021 shut down most of Texas as the power grids folded under extreme temperatures and demand. I remember the darkness of the night and the one candle that we had in the house. It did not have a very big wick on it, but it had enough. The fire burned in that little candle enough to light our living room. We were able to see each other and play cards. This reminds me that even if we feel small and insignificant, we are a light. If we choose to shine, our light carries further than we realize. Hiding under a bushel does no good for anyone. Let your light shine. Because YES!

14. Today, try to be better than you were yesterday.

Despite my best efforts, I fall short sometimes. I have kids, but nobody trains you to be a parent. I know that I make mistakes. I am married, but I've had no formal training on how to be a wife. Sometimes I fear that I am not doing enough in my marriage or in my family. Every day, though, I try to be better than I was yesterday. When I fail, I ask for forgiveness. I have learned to accept that only a flower grows quietly and that in this life, we make mistakes. I simply look in the mirror and give myself grace. Tomorrow is a new day, and each new day holds new possibilities. Be nice to yourself when you fail and try to be better tomorrow than you were today. Because YES!

15. Get out of the boat and keep your eyes on Jesus.

If you want to walk on water, you've got to get out of the boat. In the Bible (Matthew 14: 22-33) there is a story about Jesus walking on water. Did you know that Peter also walked on water? Peter started to sink when he took his eyes off Jesus. Peter trusted enough to get out of the boat, but when the doubt started to creep in, Peter took his eyes off Jesus- and began to sink. Don't be like Peter. In this life, you must sometimes get out of the boat in order to do extraordinary things. Do not let doubt and fear creep in though. Keep your eyes on Jesus. Because YES!

16. Tuesdays are the best days of the week.

> Tuesdays are my favorite day of the week because they have no expectations. Monday is the first day of the week. Wednesday is "Hump Day." Thursday is the day before Friday. Friday is the end of the work week. Saturdays and Sundays are the weekend. But Tuesday is just Tuesday. Travel is usually cheaper on Tuesdays. Tuesdays are for Tacos and that's just about it. I like Tuesday because it is the most normal feeling day of the week. Because YES!

17. Always have the next thing booked.

> We all need something to look forward to. I enjoy traveling and doing new things. I find that I am most productive when I have something to look forward to. I use Priceline to book trips- even if I must end up cancelling them. When the kids were little, I was fearful to commit to anything. Now, I book trips with the "free cancellation" and "pay later" options. This gives me the freedom to book the trip without reservation and to change my mind if something comes up. I always have something in my "upcoming trips" queue- even if I'm not sure exactly how it will happen. This reminds me of when I was younger and played basketball in school. My dad would say, "You will miss 100% of the shots you never took." In other words, the only way to score is to shoot the ball. You might miss, but you'll never score points unless you take the shot. The same is true for our trips. Most of the time, we end up going. I've only cancelled twice and once was only because something better came up. Because YES!

18. "Whether you think you can or you can't- you're right." - Henry Ford

> Your thoughts are your reality. I've become quite good at hearing what other people tell themselves. It can be quite disappointing when you begin to hear how poorly we talk to ourselves. I have mentioned this idea in a few other YESisms, but I wanted you to know that you are right. Whatever you think, you're right. Your

reality is just that- your reality. It doesn't mean that you are right; it means that what you think is what you believe to be right. If you think you can't afford something, then you can't. But you can. You can afford whatever you want, but you'll have to sacrifice something else. You can absolutely go to Disney World, but your car might get repossessed. You can absolutely get a new purse, but your kids might get tired of Ramen. You can quit drinking. You can quit overeating. You can quit making excuses and take back your life. You are the boss of yourself. You get to decide. Whatever you decide- is your reality. Because YES!

19. Thanksgiving dinner doesn't have to be in November.

Why do we wait until the fourth Thursday in November to give thanks? Why do we only eat turkey, dressing, green bean casserole, and cranberry sauce once a year? Do you like turkey and dressing? Great! Make it on the second Tuesday in February- Because YES! Don't wait. You can have Thanksgiving dinner any day of the week. You can celebrate people on days that are not their birthday! I have a friend who loves birthday cake. She'll get a day-old cake from the bakery and have "Happy Unbirthday Henry" written on it for no good reason. She doesn't even know anyone named Henry. It doesn't matter. If you like cake, get cake and pick someone to celebrate. Make tacos on Saturday if you like tacos- you do not have to wait for Tuesdays to come back around. Give yourself permission to do things differently and/or out of order. Because YES!

20. "I'm so glad we did" feels so much better than "I wish we would have."

On a whim, I found round-trip airfare to New York for dirt cheap. My sister, brother-in-law, my husband, and I flew to NYC on a Saturday afternoon. We shared a hotel overlooking Broadway, ate dinner in Times Square, took in a comedy show, toured the 9/11 museum, and flew home on Sunday night for less than

$200 each. We joked about going and then just booked the trip less than three hours before departing. We've often talked about that trip and how good it felt to go. My mom and dad keep saying, "I wish we would have gone." Yep. There it is. Don't do that. If you have a chance to go somewhere or do something, do it. Don't hesitate or list a bunch of reasons why you shouldn't or can't. Make the decision to go the next time someone asks you to lunch. Just go. At least give yourself permission to ask, "In 10 years… will I regret going or will I regret not going?" Because YES!

21. People that make time in their lives for things they enjoy-enjoy life.

We've talked about doing more things that you enjoy. Make the time. When you see people enjoying their life, it is because they've made the time to do things they enjoy. There's really no secret to life. The secret is that there is no secret- only choices. You get to choose how you spend your days. Think about the things you enjoy and do those things more often. I'm not encouraging you to quit your job and go fishing, but if you enjoy fishing, make the time to go more often. You don't have to have a fishing guide, a big boat, and a whole weekend. Grab a pole and head to your local community pond. Use a lure and cast a few times. Even if you don't catch anything, you were still by the water with a pole in the pond. You were fishing. Fishing is never really about the fish anyway- those are a bonus. If you love shopping, stop at a store. You don't have to buy anything. Making a purchase is a bonus. If you enjoy quilting but don't have a sewing machine, draw and color a design on graph paper. It isn't rocket science. If you make more time for things that you enjoy in life, you will enjoy life more. It really is that simple. Make the time. Because YES!

22. But, did you die?

Oh, gosh. I may get in trouble for this YESism. You know, it's just true. Sometimes there are times when you just have to go for it. You might win; you might lose. Either way, you'll learn. I was at a funeral for a friend's dad not too long ago. Our kids were little. We were sitting with another couple, and we were talking about sliding into home plate during a baseball game. Our friend's son yelled, "But, did you die?" We were so embarrassed because clearly someone had died, but it resonated with me to my core. Life is about taking risks. No, you shouldn't do things that are super dangerous and inflict pain on your body, but we should teach our kids (and often ourselves) to go for it! If you know the risks and you have a chance to go for it, then run like the dickens and slide into home! If you always live in fear, you're still going to die. If you take the risk, what is the worst that can happen? I mean, I don't want you to die. I don't want to die. But I'd rather die doing what I love and living free than live with fear and regret. After all, what good is life if you don't live? What would be the point? Don't be dumb. This is not giving you permission to tempt fate, but don't be so caught up in the what-ifs and the reasons why you should not do something. Make a decision and go for it! No regrets. Make good choices- and don't die. Because YES!

23. Today is the day!

Carpe diem! Seize the day! You and I are not guaranteed tomorrow. We can make plans, and we can want to do something, but the only thing we can be certain of is change. Things change. People change. If you need to let go of fear, resentment, doubt, worry, or any other baggage, today is the day. Let it go. If you need to apologize to someone, do it. If you need to forgive someone, do it. If you need to repent, do it. If you've never invited Jesus into your heart, today is the day. Don't wait. You may never get another chance to tell someone you love them. You may never get the chance to make the call. I know it's not easy to reach out, but the longer you wait, the less likely you are to do it. I don't know what it is, but if there is something tugging at you, just handle it. Handle it and let it go.

You CAN do it. You are worthy of happiness, and we all have things we need to let go. Today is the day. Because YES!

24. Say what you want out loud. Tell others- they'll help you find it.

Do not be afraid to say what you want. Say it out loud. Many self-help gurus talk about the importance of writing things down. I agree that writing things down can have profound therapeutic effects. Albert Einstein once said, "A thought not written down is just a dream." I agree, but I have found that saying things out loud has power. Verbalizing your desires sends energy into the Universe and the Universe responds. For example, I was in Cancun in 2021. I asked the taxi driver to stop at the CANCUN sign because I wanted to take a picture on top of it. He said he didn't know where the sign I showed him was. As soon as we arrived at the market, though, there was a similar CANCUN sign, and I got my picture. Then, at the airport, my son helped me find yet another CANCUN sign. I took another picture! I believe that you should say what you want and tell others. People want to help you accomplish your goals and live your dreams. With saying that, listen to people. Oftentimes, people will tell you what they want, need, or desire if you simply stop and listen. Help them reach their goals and find what they are looking for. Because YES!

25. Make the plate.

In the South, making a plate for someone at mealtimes is a way of showing honor and respect. My grandmother always fixed my grandfather a plate. I thought it was such an outdated practice and often asked her about it. She would just tell me that one day I would understand. I saw my mom make my dad's plate many times. Not as much as my grandma, but almost always at dinner. She also packed him a lunch. I vowed to marry someone that made me a plate. What I found, though, was I enjoy making my husband's plate. I, too, make his lunch. I do not do it because I have to, and I don't make his plate every night. I make my husband's plate because it feels good to do something for someone else. I enjoy serving him in this way. I might be old-fashioned, but I have learned that by serving him dinner, I am telling him that I love him. It's kind of silly when I read this, but it is my truth. I appreciate the mutual respect and honor we share. I am not my husband's servant, but we are partners, and taking care of each other is important. A little act of kindness goes a long way. Guess what? My husband makes my plate, too. We work in tandem. I include this little YESism as a suggestion, but it is more than making someone's plate. Serving others feels good. When we share responsibility, serve one another, and seek ways to honor each other, our relationships grow. Never let pride or society's prejudice interfere with your ability to serve. You are not lesser if you put others first- you are actually selfless. Because YES!

26. Stay ahead of the mouse.

One of the most interesting and profound discussions I have with students is when we talk about priorities. There is a free game online called "MouseTrap." The object of the game is to trap the mouse. I win just about every single time I play. I have learned how to trap the mouse. You start by placing pillars around the perimeter of the game board. Each time you place a pillar, though, the mouse moves. Usually, the mouse will move in the opposite direction of where you want him to go. Thus, you put the pillars opposite of where you think he will go and begin closing him in. The crazy thing is that many people get frustrated with the mouse and blame the mouse for being smarter than them. The mouse is always looking for the path of least resistance. You know the minute the mouse beats you and it is best to let it go and restart. The same is true for life. The only way to win is to stay ahead of the mouse. Anticipate the barriers to your success and work to succeed. There will be times that the mouse wins. Let it go. Restart. Cry if you need to, but just let it go. You can't change the outcome once the mouse gets ahead. Don't quit playing just because you lost a round. Restart and celebrate when you do win. Set your pillars around the perimeter and work backwards. Move. Adjust. Stay ahead of the mouse. Because YES!

27. Flip-flops = Walking feet.

The doctors told us that our son, Taylin, would never sit, stand, or walk. I struggled with this for years. When Taylin was about 14 months old, he was fitted for his first pair of braces for his feet. I'll never forget that experience. We had to go to a prosthetics clinic and have molds of his feet made so they could custom make his braces. I cried. I remember thinking that since he had braces, he could never wear flip-flops. I cried. I love flip-flops. I quit wearing flip-flops, though, because I felt that it was unfair to wear them in front of him. I failed to see that the braces were strengthening his feet and ankles so that he could walk. Walking with braces was still walking- even if the braces only fit inside of tennis shoes. A few years later, Taylin began walking without the braces. He wore strong, supportive high-top tennis shoes for a while, but eventually, he began walking in normal shoes. We have a pool in the backyard, so he started wearing Crocs. I never will forget the day he came out to the pool in flip-flops. I guess he couldn't find his Crocs, so he just wore his sister's flip-flops. I cried. This time, I cried because he was wearing flip-flops and walking. For years now, flip-flops have served to remind me that nothing is impossible with God. Walking feet are both physical and metaphorical for me. Every time you see flip-flops, I encourage you to stop and say, "Thank you!" for walking feet. By the way, June 18th is National Flip-Flop Day in America! Because YES!

28. Say YES to filters.

When cell phones first came out, I had the pink Razor flip phone. I loved that phone. I didn't want a fancy iPhone or any of the bells and whistles. I did want a phone that took good pictures. I have since upgraded, but I still don't have a fancy phone with all the bells and whistles. My kids do, though. My daughters are obsessed with filters. I fought the good fight and finally waved the white flag and took a picture with a filter. Oh. My. Gosh! I looked 10 years younger and much thinner. My make-up was suddenly perfect. YES! What I learned is that it is okay to use a filter if you know who you are. Don't use a filter if you think you must. You are beautiful and perfect the way you are. Occasionally, though, it is fun to see yourself through a different lens. Because YES!

29. Line dancing and back roads are good for the soul.

I grew up in a little farming town in the middle of North Texas. Literally, I grew up across from a cornfield. I learned to drive on the back roads. I love driving, and nothing is better than a dirt road in the middle of nowhere. If you find yourself needing a break from reality, I suggest you grab a Big Red and Moon Pie and head out of the rat race. Find the nearest back road and drive. Drive until your shoulders begin to relax. Roll down the windows and smell the fresh air. Then, pull over and turn up your radio. In the middle of nowhere, play "Copper Head Road" and do a line dance. Laugh. Smile. Sing. Mess up. Keep dancing in the middle of nowhere like nobody is watching. Because YES!

30. People are good.

I still believe people are good. Some people are bad, and I get that. There are dangerous people in this world. But I still believe that most people are good. I went fishing last summer off the coast of Texas. My son wanted to fish, and I had absolutely no gear. To make matters worse, I was alone because my husband was working on the island where we were staying. In true YES! fashion, though, I agreed. My son and I rented poles and headed out to the dock. I didn't think things all the way through, though, because before I knew it, my son had hooked a fish. Excellent! And, Yikes! What was I going to do? I hadn't thought about what to do if we actually caught a fish. I asked this nice gentleman if he could help us take off the fish, and he was more than happy to do so. He was a retired Marine and was out fishing with his family. This guy spent the entire morning helping us bait, cast, and take fish off our lines. He wouldn't accept any payment, and he had just as much fun helping us as he did helping his own family. I was reminded that most people are good. I could go on and on about how the goodness of others has impacted our lives. We have been blessed beyond measure, and I am honored to be able to pay it forward in any way we can. I try to be over the top excited about finding ways to help others, and I try to give people the benefit of the doubt. Don't ever lose faith in the goodness of others. Be a good person. Yield the right of way. Slow down. Extend grace. Be the reason why someone else smiles. Remind someone else that there are still good people by being a good person. Offer to help take someone else's fish off the hook, and don't be afraid to ask for help. There are still really great people out there. Be one of them. Because YES!

31. Find abundance through intentional play.

I have a love/hate relationship with money. They say money cannot buy you happiness, but let's be honest. Money allows you to do things and buy things that you enjoy. I have changed my outlook on spending and saving money. I'm still pretty responsible, but I have learned to trust that money is just paper energy. I have studied my own belief systems by reading "Mastering Affluence" by Carrol Tuttle and by participating in a 30-day money game. My friend, Jeanie King, leads a 30-day money game in which participants begin to spend money each day on things they want, need, and desire. By "playing" with money, you learn to release your inhibitions and just enjoy the thought of spending freely. The strangest thing has happened, though. Each time I have played the game, I find that my trust and understanding of money as energy is enlightened. I can bend, mold, and flex my financial muscles. I have learned that I not only have enough, I have plenty. I am rich in love, relationships, knowledge, and even finances. I have everything I need and most of what I want. I have learned that what I cannot afford is a lie. This book is not about finding financial freedom but learning to question your belief systems and changing the idea that you cannot afford something is essential. If you struggle with money, I encourage you to connect with Jeanie King (https://www.linkedin.com/in/jeanie-king-73a16839/). Because YES!

32. Drink it up!

I drink a lot. It doesn't really matter what I drink, I just drink a lot. I drink a lot of water, coffee, juice, etc. I encourage you to think about how liquid enters our bodies, and hydrates us. Think about how you must bring the cup to your mouth, swallow it, and refill it as much as you can. The same is true when good things are happening. "Drink it up" is a phrase I use to encourage myself to participate in the blessings. When my daughter graduated, I drank it up. Every last drop of that senior year. I planned for and saved to be able to say YES! to everything that year. The prom dress, the shoes, the sash for cheerleading, senior breakfast, and even senior skip day… I enjoyed that time and loved watching her enjoy it, too! I think it is super important to recognize the good times and to give yourself permission to drink it up! Make the slurping sound! Lick the bowl- whatever you have to do to celebrate the good days, do it! Because YES!

33. 24 hours.

You have the same 24 hours every day that Michelangelo had when he painted the Sistine Chapel in Rome. Make every minute count! One of the things I hear people say is, "I don't have time" or "I wish I had more time." The truth is that we have the time we make time for. I talked about doing a time audit earlier in the book. On my website, I provide a free time audit worksheet for you to use to investigate where you spend your time. If you are honest with yourself, you can find time to do just about anything you want. I worked full-time as an elementary teacher, taught two courses online as an adjunct professor, and was a full-time doctoral student while raising three children with medical issues. I promise. If I can do it, you can, too. Be truly honest with yourself about your time. What are you doing? Really? Every minute of every day. Some people commit to three days at first. That's great. The problem is that you really need to keep account for seven straight days to see where you are spending your time- during the week and on the weekends. Are you driving too much? Can you take a different route or leave earlier to avoid traffic? Can you listen to podcasts that are encouraging during that time? Are you spending too much time on social media? (Guilty.) Start figuring out where you can grab extra minutes each day. What will you do with your extra time? Ten minutes each day equals over an hour a week. What could you do with an extra hour? What can you accomplish? You cannot bank your minutes, so each day, what can you do? If you have extra time, do something you enjoy. If you enjoy fishing (like me), can you use those bonus minutes to restring your line or organize your lures? Can you lay your boots by the back door so that you can save time later when you sneak down to the lake? What can you do? By learning to "budget" your time, you'll find that you have more than enough time to do what you must do and more time to do what you want to do. Because YES!

34. You are the boss.

I have a very poorly written, emotionally charged blog post from when my daughter experienced her back injury. I've thought about rewriting it, and maybe I will, but the truth is that my life changed when I decided to be the boss. What I mean by this is that there are things you can do right now to take ownership of your situation. You can do lots of things to help yourself. There are loads of alternative measures and holistic options for your health. I had no idea until I began to search beyond Western medicines and doctors. I learned about massage, essential oils, cryotherapy, water therapy, and even ceremonies by modern-day Shamans. I took ownership of our medical situation and started forming an action plan. I became the medical coordinator and case manager. I did the research, took notes, and scheduled appointments. Deciding I was the BOSS changed my life. Sometimes our situations feel out of control. It is up to you to declare yourself as the boss of your life. As a boss, you hire (employ) people who share your same value and mission statements. You decide when you work. You decide the direction to move- because you are the boss. Today, decide that you are the boss of your life. You make the decisions. You get to decide from this point forward what is next. You are the BOSS. Because YES!

35. Microwave. Start with the microwave.

Cleaning my house is not my specialty. I'm not very good at cleaning, and I do not enjoy all the chores associated with cleaning my house. The daunting task of housework can be paralyzing. To combat that feeling, focus on one thing: the microwave. If I can clean the microwave, then I have done one thing. When I get the microwave cleaned, I can wipe down the counter it sits on. If that counter gets wiped down and I already have the spray out, I can do the adjacent counter. If I get those two counters cleaned, then I can probably wipe down the other counters. Pretty soon, my kitchen is cleaned, and I can start on the bathrooms. If I get one bathroom cleaned, then I can move to the other one. If not, at least I got the microwave cleaned. I suppose my thinking for this YESism is that if you get overwhelmed by a large task, break it down. Start with something manageable and work from there. Give yourself grace and permission to do one thing well. It is hard to find the motivation when the tasks can seem so big. If you can just do one thing, though, then celebrate the small victory. Because YES!

36. "Be too much candy for a dime." -Jeff Steinbrenner

My dad used to say this all the time. When someone would go out of their way to help another, my dad would say, "He's just too much candy for a dime." I love that. This is a simple little reminder that you don't get much for a dime, but when you get a little extra, that's too much. I encourage all of us to try and be "too much candy for a dime." What can you do that is above and beyond what is expected? Our buddy, Ross Light, lets us fish on his property. The fish in his pond always bite, and we love spending time on the farm. When we call and ask Ross if we can come out, he's always super happy to have us. He'll take the trolling motor and oars down to the lake for us. He doesn't have to do that. He also will offer to clean the fish, let us use his RV, or help us build something if we ask. A few years ago, Jason talked about needing hinges for the gate at our house. Ross showed up and put them on for us while Jason was at work. Ross really is "too much candy for a dime!" Think of how you can be "too much candy for a dime!" Because YES!

37. Be responsible.

I've worked really hard to be spontaneous and to learn to say YES! whenever possible. Responsible behaviors, though, are part of saying YES! We have three dogs. It is difficult for me to spend the money on flea medicines and shots. Grr. I also find it difficult to pay for things like haircuts, dental work, and oil changes. Getting an inspection and paying for registration for our vehicles chaps my hide. The responsible things are often not fun to pay for. Doing the right thing, though, is always right. Have fun. Do fun things. But, be responsible for your actions. Buy the flea medicine, get the rabies shots, register your vehicle, and get your teeth cleaned. I know it's not the most fun thing in the world but be responsible. Because YES!

38. Do something because someone else wants to do it.

My parents have been married for almost 50 years. Their parents were married for over 50 years. My husband's parents were married for 50 years until death did them part, and their parents were also married for 50 plus years. We come from a long line of married folks. I've been married for almost two decades, and even though times have not always been perfect, it has been a great ride. People ask me how it works. It works because we have a lot of give and take. Let's talk about Elvis. Before I met my husband, I knew very little about Elvis Presley. Jason is obsessed with Elvis. Every year we make an annual pilgrimage to Graceland in Memphis, Tennessee. Jason tours the house and goes to all the museums. Me, not so much. I did it one year, and every once in a while, I'll go on the tours, but I'd rather hang out at the pool. I go to the concerts, and I enjoy being with Jason. Elvis is not really my thing, but Jason is. He enjoys the music, the memories, the fans, and the feeling of being in Memphis. So, we go, and we sing, and we have fun. The same is true for the beach. I love the beach. Jason cannot stand the sand and the sun, so he'll grab a chair and umbrella and drag the cooler down to the water. He'll sit and listen to Elvis on the radio while we play in the waves. It's not his thing, but I am. So, he goes, and smiles, and has a good time. The thing about relationships is that there are times when you do things just because it is what the other person likes. It might not be your thing but do it anyway. And don't do things because you have to. Do things because you know that your partner enjoys them, and you enjoy being with your partner. Have fun for real- don't just pretend. Allow yourself to shake, rattle and roll! If you can't beat them, join them! Wear the jumpsuit, blue suede shoes, and say, "Thank you. Thank you very much." Because YES!

39. Say "NO."

Okay, I know this sounds weird because we are focusing on saying YES- but saying YES means saying NO to things that are not good for you. That means that you should give yourself permission to step back from things that take away your time, focus, and energy. For instance, if you find that you do not have time for fishing because you volunteer too much, then step back from your volunteering. Yes, you love volunteering, but you also love fishing. There must be a balance. I love social media, but I also have two jobs and a family. I do not allow myself to participate on social media until I have done what I must do for my work and family. Sometimes I sneak in a scroll before making dinner, but usually, I put down my computer and phone so that I can focus on real-life facetime. Saying "NO" to things allows you the time and energy to say "YES!" to time and energy focusing on what you really want. Another example is to examine your finances. My checking account online will break my spending into categories. I found that our expenses for eating out were greater than our grocery bill. This meant that we were spending way too much on going out to eat rather than eating at home. Eating out does not align to our core values of time at home, healthy cooking, and saving money. So, we made a conscious decision to stop eating out as much, which saves us money to use for doing more fun things than grabbing a burger on the way home from work. We say YES! to the things we value. Because YES!

40. Get up early. Make your bed.

Admiral William H. McRaven wrote "Make Your Bed: Little Things That Can Change Your Life." This book solidified my thoughts about making your bed every morning. Admiral McRaven explained that as a Navy Seal, the first act of the morning is to make your bed with razor-sharp precision. This one act was perfected each day, so much so that it became second nature. There was no choice but to make your bed daily, and not just make the bed, but make it well. That way, as the last act of the day, you can get into your well-made bed and be comforted in the knowledge that even if the day had been a train wreck, at least you were ending it in a well-made bed. I've always made my bed- even before reading the book. I don't always make it perfectly like a Navy Seal, but I do straighten the covers so that it looks presentable. My friend, Joyce, used to laugh at this because I can have dishes stacked in the sink and nine million loads of laundry waiting to be folded, but by goodness by golly, my bed is made. You might find it funny that I do not have a flat sheet on our bed. I love a flat sheet on my bed, but when there is a flat sheet on the bed, my husband and I fight over it and the comforter. Inevitably, one of us wakes up with a sheet and one with the comforter. We decided early in our marriage that it wasn't worth it. We only sleep with a comforter unless we are at a hotel where the sheets are already on the bed. And, even though we have pillow shams and throw pillows for the bed, we only put those on when guests are coming over. Otherwise, making the bed really is just about straightening the comforter and putting the remotes on the nightstand. Whatever you have to do to make things work, just do it. If nothing else, just straighten your comforter like me. It takes less than a minute, and at the end of the day, at least you can smile at your efforts. Because YES!

41. Give yourself grace.

I'm not a great housekeeper. and I've stopped trying to live up to the expectations I used to set for myself. I am not great at saving money. I am really hard on myself, and I used to let my circumstances and situations control me. I thought that because I stayed home with Taylin when he was a baby, I was supposed to somehow become a super mom in a traditional domestic role. I would get up early and make Jason breakfast. Dinner would be on the table when he got home. I was working harder than I had ever worked in my life while I stayed home. I was still working online as an adjunct professor and running a junking business. For some reason, I still felt that because I was "at home," I should be doing all the things that I perceived as my chores. Ridiculous. Looking back, I remember having so much resentment and honor at the same time. I felt like I was honoring my husband and family by serving in the little wifey role. I was so resentful, though, that my husband got to get up and go to work. He got a break. He didn't have to deal with the medical doctors, medicine issues, scheduling, insurance, therapies, and all the things that come with having a special needs kid. He didn't have to go to the grocery store and try to make dinners for a family of 5 for under $10. He didn't have to do one dish or clean a toilet or take out the trash. I did it all. I even mowed most of the time so that I could just enjoy spending time with him when he was home. How dumb. I was so frustrated and exhausted when he got home that I didn't want to be around him- and he hadn't even done anything to provoke my anger. I had to learn to be nice to myself. It took a few years, and I'm probably still too hard on myself, but I have learned to let things go. I am also better at asking for help. If I don't get to the dishes, someone else will- or they won't. It's okay. I have learned to look past lots of things that I used to get twisted up over. The only person I hurt was myself, and I find that my husband really doesn't mind doing things with me. He doesn't mind doing the dishes or taking out the trash or whatever needs to be done. He also doesn't mind if things don't get done. I encourage you to be nice to yourself. Give yourself grace. Learn to look past the dishes in the sink and just be grateful for the food you ate off them. Be thankful for the feet that wear the basket of unfolded socks in your living room. Let it go and know that in this season, you may not get to everything you think you should. Grace. And, for goodness sake, don't judge others who give themselves grace. There are way more important things than a perfect house and matching socks. Because YES!

42. Be in the pictures.

For years, I was absent from our pictures. I took the pictures and was happy to be behind the camera instead of in front of it. Let's be honest: I was embarrassed by the way I looked. If I was in a picture, I pulled one of the kids in front of me so that you couldn't see anything except for my head. Ridiculous. My friend called me out on it a while back. She said that nobody cares about how you look. Your kids will look at the pictures and remember how much fun you had together, and you want to be in their memories. I'm better now. I find that I started to be in the pictures more often, and it is nice. I have lost about 60 lbs. and being in pictures now isn't nearly as painful as it was, but even when I was much heavier, I started being in the pictures. Fine. Just know that if you hide in every picture, there's a missed opportunity to be in the memories. Your kids deserve you to be present- now and in the future. Be in the pictures. Because YES!

43. Laugh.

Just laugh. If you don't know how, go to laughing yoga. If there's not a laughing yoga class near you, Google it. It's ridiculous, I know. But the truth is that your body does not know the difference between real laughter and the act of laughing. Lots of studies have been done concerning the use of laughter therapy to combat medical problems. The results have been exponentially encouraging. There are no negative effects of laughter- except if you pee a little when you laugh (thanks menopause!). Sometimes as adults, we forget to laugh genuinely and without reservation. You may not have the time to sit down and focus on your laughter but make it a point to find humor in situations. Do fun things on purpose and surround yourself with people who laugh. If you aren't funny, look up funny things. There is a whole YouTube channel devoted to making you laugh. Read funny stories or joke books if you need to. It is hard to remember to laugh- especially when nothing seems or feels funny. I know there are many times when laughter is not the first reaction to a situation or when it feels wrong. Try to laugh anyway. If you have to, fake it. Remember, the body does not know the difference between real and perceived laughter. You get the same benefits, so just laugh. Say out loud, "Ha, Ha, Hahaha!" Say it again in a lion's voice, "HAARR, HAAR, HAAARRRHAAARRRR HARRRR!" Because YES!

44. Practice NOW.

I beg you to practice being happy now- today- in this moment. Practice building your neuropathways to happiness like it is the most important thing you have on your plate. Practice your calming techniques, practice your breathing, practice your tapping, meridian pressure points, self-talking, prioritization of the moments, and task orientation meditation. Life is most certainly going to throw you curve balls and threaten your homeostasis. If you are not equipped to handle the stress, you will more than likely fall back into your old habits of thought and stress. It is normal to accept your circumstances and think negatively- but it is not okay. You are better than that. You are wonderfully and perfectly crafted and designed for more than a life of mediocracy, worry, doubt, and fear. You are equipped with the ability to take control over your mind, body, and circumstances- but you need to take advantage of today- right now- start learning and investing in yourself. Because YES!

45. There is no shame in asking for help- including online grocery shopping.

When the COVID-19 pandemic hit, people were crazy about hoarding groceries. I remember going to the grocery store an hour and a half before it opened just so that I could be one of the first ones in. I would gather what we needed and be gone. I would often buy things we didn't really need in case we needed them at some point. Ridiculous. I even made a make-shift pantry in my bedroom for our overstocked and non-perishable items. Then, as life began to get back to normal, I stopped going to the grocery store as often and started going back to my list days. I found that I spent more time thinking about what I needed than I did grocery shopping. Then, I discovered grocery delivery. I had come down with COVID-19, so I had no choice but to have groceries delivered. It was so easy to open the website, select what I needed, and then voila! Groceries appeared on my doorstep. What I realized is that groceries cost a little extra to have delivered, but I did not buy random stuff. I was able to save time and money by being nice to myself and asking for help. I had no idea just how much time I was saving until I went back to the store. My weekly grocery adventures were 2-3 hours long. That was about 10-12 hours per month of just grocery shopping. Now, it takes me about 10-15 minutes, and my grocery fairy delivers. The point is that you may not even know that you need help. Ask for help and see how it goes. You may not need groceries delivered, but you might just find that you save time and money by soliciting services you don't think you need. Groceries, cleaning, yard work, etc… what can you invest in that will ultimately help you achieve your bigger goals? Try asking for help. Because YES!

46. Be nice to yourself.

All the self-help and personal growth books will encourage you to be aware of your relationship with yourself. Watch how you talk to yourself and about yourself. Yada, Yada, Yada. I remember rolling my eyes at myself as I was learning how to become a better version of myself. I am still perfecting this YESism in my personal life, but we really should make an effort to be nice to ourselves. If you are like me, I struggled with so many things, and working on my relationship with myself was always left on the back burner. I started slowly. I started to take a bath again at night with a splash of "Sleep" lavender oil from Bath and

Body Works. I had been using a little of my oils sparingly from time to time, but I decided to start making bath time about me. I purchased a new bottle of sleep bath oils, lotion, and spray for my pillow. Baths became a nightly routine of how I began being nice to myself. While in the bath, I started trying these affirmation statements that the books talked about. I started with saying things like, "You kept the tiny humans alive today. Good job." And "You didn't screw up too bad or burn dinner. Good job." Pretty soon, I realized that these were not at all affirmative-they were just recognizing that I didn't suck as a mom, wife, or woman. I started trying to think of other things to say to myself. I started working my way into "You are a good mom. You care about people. You are worthy. You deserve to be happy. This is only the beginning." As I started saying nice things to myself, I started to believe them. It may have only been bath time routines, but I began investing a little more into myself. Pretty soon, an email came across my mailbox offering tuition discounts for the doctoral program at my university. That night, I took a bath and thought, "You are worthy. You are smart. You are capable." I applied the next day and started that summer working on my doctorate degree. Don't get me wrong, I am still my worst critic, but I have stopped being so hard on myself. I do nice things for myself, and I am more conscious of how I speak to and about myself. We're all a work in progress. Because YES!

47. Learn to receive compliments.

This is a funny YESism for me to explain. It seems straightforward enough, right? So, why is it difficult for us to accept compliments? For me, I find it easier to refuse a compliment by denying what has been said. For example, when someone says, "Your hair looks great today!" I usually say something like, "Thanks! I washed it for the first time in three days." Or, even worse is when I say something like, "I know right? Usually it looks like crap!" WHY? WHY do we do that? Just say, "Thank you!" If you can, reply with a genuine compliment, or just leave it at thank you. I have become much better at accepting compliments, and in turn, am able to genuinely compliment others. Accepting compliments allows us to receive the goodness and appreciation shown to us by others. Because YES!

48. Find the time.

Yes- YOU- find the time to do things you enjoy. You have the time; you just might not know it. Like saving money or dieting, finding time takes discipline. Do the work. We talked about having the same 24 hours a day as everyone else. We've talked about being nice to yourself and about having no excuses. This YESism is about finding the time. Can you minimize your make-up routine in the morning? I minimized my everyday make-up routine to include six items: wearing base, powder, blush, eyeshadow, mascara, and lipstick. I bought two sets of the same six items, and I keep one set in my desk drawer and the other one on my vanity. If I dress up, I have my "good" make-up in a different drawer, but for everyday purposes, I have streamlined the process. The time I save may only be minutes each day, but if I save 10 minutes a day, that is over an hour a week- just by adjusting my make-up routine. That gives me an extra hour each week to do something I want to do. You can find the time. What can you streamline to afford you more time to do the things you want to do? What can you do with an extra hour each week? Find the time. Because YES!

49. Seasons.

Remember that you are in a "Season." I'm not sure what "Season" you are in, but try to enjoy it. I was in the Season of Babies for a while. I was in the Season of Medical Hell. I have been in the Season of Diagnosis After Diagnosis, Surgeries, and Therapy. I am currently in a new Season of Graduation and High School adventures. Crazy enough, I am also in the Season of Elementary Parties and Valentine

Exchanges with my son. There is joy in all of the seasons, but they also come with challenges. Try to remember that this moment is a season. The diaper changes will soon be exchanged for swim lessons. The swim lessons will transition into sleepovers. Those sleepovers will turn into awkward hairstyles, social media training, and those mouths will speak in ways that will leave you scratching your head. If you find that you are frustrated by a season, just hang on. Seasons change. And, if you are enjoying the season, drink it up! Because YES!

50. When the beach calls, answer with YES!!!!

I love the beach. I love the way the air smells and feels on my skin. I love the constant breeze and the way the saltwater buffs my skin. I love walking on the sand and feeling the sun beat down on my shoulders to the point where it stings a little. I like the way my skin looks with a sun kiss and how exfoliated I feel after a cool shower and some aloe vera. More than anything, I love how free I feel when I stand in awe of the majestic waves and exponential power that exists beyond my control. I look out into the ocean, and I remember just how little my life is in comparison to the world that encompasses me. When I am feeling super overwhelmed, I find that a trip to the beach grounds me. I remember talking to my daughter when she was just about to enter her senior year of high school. She was facing some difficult situations with friends, and I did the one thing I knew to do. I took her to the beach. In the middle of chasing the waves on our boogie board, I paused, grabbed her shoulders, and turned her body to face down the beach. I explained that as far as your eyes can see, not one person cares who your friends are, what your degree is, or what grade you make in school. The people that are with you care about you. This big world can swallow you up in two seconds if you start thinking that your problems are bigger than God. Being at the beach reminds me just how small we are and how big God is. He doesn't want us to be overwhelmed and consumed by the world. Instead, we should look out onto the waves, enjoy the sunrise, and bask in His glory. Soak up the sun. Walk barefoot. Catch a fish. Laugh. Surf. Forget your problems and head to the ocean. On one of my last trips to the beach, I tried meaningful meditation. The idea is to sit quietly and not think, just listen. The position of receiving is to sit with your palms up and be still. I tried doing this by walking out to the end of the jetty. I sat in the spot where the waves crash around and splash up just enough to tickle my toes. I sat quietly and reverently with my palms up while I prayed and tried to clear my mind. The sound of the waves and the breeze in my hair felt so amazing. I am not good at sitting still, but the sound of waves crashing stilled my soul. I opened myself up to the blessings around me, and I remember feeling rested for the first time in a long while. Any time you get a chance to go to the beach, go. When you are feeling overwhelmed, go. When you are not feeling overwhelmed, go. If only in your mind, go. Head straight into the sun, look over the horizon, and marvel at His majestic wonder. Be still. Put your palms to the sky and sit in quiet reverence. Listen to the sound of the ocean and let the waves calm your mind. Because YES!

51. Live without regrets.

In ten years, what will you regret more, doing it or not doing it? When you're trying to decide, think about the results of your decision in 10 years. Will you regret going or not going? Will you regret spending the money? If your answer has to do with money, let it go. Money comes and goes. I'm not giving you permission to spend your last dollar; I'm simply encouraging you to improve your relationship with money. If you are trying to decide what to do, ask yourself the 10-year question. What will your future self thank you for? Will you wish you would have gone? Will you wish you would have quit that job? Will you wish that you had spent more time at work? Make good decisions and when you have the chance, go for it. Because YES!

52. Wait for it ... Patience is a virtue...

My cousins took me ice fishing last year. The first thing you do is cut a rectangular hole in the ice about 3 feet x 2 feet. Then, you drag the fish house over the hole. The fish house has a hole in the bottom of it and has benches on each side. It is pitch black in the fish house, but the sun off the snow and ice illuminates the bottom of the lake and lights up the whole house. You use a little decoy and a baitfish. You move the little decoy around and sit patiently. You hold a spear that looks like a pitchfork over your shoulder and wait until a Northern Pike creeps into the vision hole. As soon as you see the fish, you drop the spear into the lake slowly, and then BAM! You release the spear with all your might and then pull like crazy. The fish comes up the hole, and you open the fish house door, put the fish out on the ice, and slam the door. The door slamming helps the fish detach from the spear, and then you can just go out and see your bounty. It is a rush! I loved ice fishing, and I have thought a lot about the experience. You sit and wait until just the right moment, and then with all your might, you thrust every bit of your strength down onto the fish. Life can be like that. You must be patient. Wait for it. Plan and prepare. Then, strike at just the right moment. Set yourself up in a position that is just right, cut the ice just right, hold the spear just right, and have a plan for what happens when you spear the fish. So, with love, I ask you to put yourself in a position to strike. Be patient. Wait for it. Be still. Be ready. There will be a fish that lurches into your hole, and you will need to be in position to grab it. Wait for it. Because YES!

53. Change your story.

You control the narrative from this point forward. If you don't like the ending, choose something different. I used to love those choose your own adventure books. The kind where if you wanted A to happen, you turned to page 32. If you wanted B to happen, you turned to page 47. Each choice led to a different outcome. The same is true with your life. You get to decide which direction you take next. If you don't like the direction you are headed, change it. Pick a different path. You get to be the author of your story. You have always had this power; you may just not have known how powerful you are. If you look back at your life and realize that you have been reactive, like I had been, then stop. Take it back. You are the boss. From this very moment, look at each new day as an opportunity to change your narrative. If you are not living in the first person, change it. Use your story to build the next chapter. Write your own storybook adventure. Choose your characters carefully. What is your setting? What's next in your playbook? Decide right now to write the best doggone adventure possible can so that when you get to the end, you will look back and say, "What an adventure!" Because YES!

54. Don't be dumb.

I tell my kids this all the time. I'm full of adventure and YES! has become a way of life for me. But don't be dumb. If you don't like your job, design an exit plan. Don't quit your job without enough money or another job to take its place. Try your best to exit wisely with integrity. Don't burn bridges. Don't drink and drive. Make a plan. I didn't say not to drink- I just said that if you know you're going to drink, don't be dumb. Go on vacation but spend your money wisely. Don't get caught up in dime store junk and souvenirs. I mean, if that's your thing, then do it. But, very rarely have we gone somewhere and returned with souvenirs. Instead, invest in the pictures and experiences. You don't need another magnet and spoon- unless you really do love those things. Otherwise, save the money and go to another museum or theme park. Another tip is to order water at dinner. You do not need iced tea or soda when you go out. Save $3 a person for the next adventure.

Little changes add up to big results. Don't be dumb. Because YES!

55. Always Up!

This piece of advice comes from years of training and work with Dr. Rich Allen. Dr. Allen allowed me to contribute to his educational books over a decade ago. The books focused on ways to engage learners through novelty, music, questioning, and movement. I loved working on these books. Moreover, I loved watching Dr. Allen present workshops for educators. In his workshop, he stressed the idea and importance of Always Up! He insisted that the classroom is a stage, and we are responsible for the mood and tone of our performance. If you have upbeat music playing and begin with a personal anecdote, you set the tone for a fun, lively, exciting workshop, or lesson. He used the example of leading a workshop in Japan where he started by putting all the chairs in rows, introducing himself, and starting a PowerPoint. After lunch, he had all the chairs stacked, had upbeat music playing, and as people walked in, he shook their hands and welcomed the executives back. They grabbed a chair and bopped along to the beat, found a seat, and he began with a story. Immediately, the tone of the room changed. Why? Because he was up. He was engaged. When you are with others, it is important to be up! I know it isn't easy to be always up, but remember that your attitude toward whatever you are doing sets the tone for what is happening. Your kids are watching. Your family is watching. Your friends, students, colleagues, etc… You may not feel up, but you should fake it until you make it. If you're in a bad mood, fine. You can stay in a bad mood, but remember your bad mood sets the tone. If you step in dog poop on the way to class, have a flat tire along the road, and your coffee is cold when you pull into the parking lot (all have happened in one morning recently for me), you can go in smelling and feeling like poop- but really that is how the day will continue to go for you if you don't make the choice to get back up. Always up. As much as you can stand it, get up. Stay up. Because YES!

56. Prep a little.

Do you know where it would be if you put it back where it belongs? It would be wherever it was supposed to be. Substitute it for whatever it is that you have misplaced. Start with putting things where they need to be. That's easier said than done when you live with little monsters who haven't learned to master the art of putting things back in their place. The first part of this YESism is that everything has a place and everything in its place saves time in the long run. The other part of this YESism is that to save time and energy, you should prep a little. For instance, my son always loses his shoes. So, his school shoes go on the TV stand in the living room. We also lay out his clothes for the next day there. No questions, just put the clothes out. This saves time in the morning. I've done this with all my kids. We pick out our clothes for the week, fold them together (or hang them up together), and stick to the plan. When Holly was cheerleading, her uniform, shoes, socks, and bow were hung together using a hanger and zip lock bag over the hanger. Same with our show clothes for livestock adventures. Shoes, jeans, shirt, belt, and the FFA t-shirt hang together. The staff shirts I have to wear on certain days stay on the back of my closet door. I always know where they are. Do yourself a favor and prep a little. Lay out your clothes, shoes, and accessories. Same is true for groceries. If you spend a little time thinking about what you need for the week, you can plan meals and get everything you need before the week begins. This saves your time and energy by knowing what you are going to need and having things ready. You won't have to decide what to make for dinner every night because you have a plan. Plan your meals around your life. What are you doing? Do you have time for a lot of prep? Who is going to be home? All these questions help you to make and plan for a successful week where you know what you are going to eat. Sure, there are times when you have leftovers or "fend for yourself" meals, but you can plan for those to. If you need a simple guide, I try to do some sort of pasta on Monday, Tuesdays are for tacos or Mexican, Wednesdays are grill out or crockpot days, Thursdays are left over days or "fend for yourself," and Fridays are pizza or go out days. The weekend plans depend on what is going on. Fend for yourself days include things like hot pockets, corn dogs, macaroni and cheese, ravioli, soups, grilled cheese sandwiches, Ramen, or anything else that is easy enough for the kids to make for themselves if they don't want leftovers. I don't always stick to this plan, but it is a generic blueprint for ideas when I am planning meals for the week. Whatever it is that you plan, be nice to yourself and prep a little. A little bit of preparation yields more time for things you enjoy doing. Because YES!

57. Send the kids away.

Oh, man. Cleaning the house while kids are home is like brushing your teeth while eating Oreos. I remember the good ol' days when my mom would send us out of the house and tell us we couldn't come back for at least two hours. I get it. I have been guilty of sending my kids out to play, too. I mean, I can see them outside, but I make my kids get out when I am cleaning. Don't feel bad if you need to take a few hours to yourself and spend time in your space. Hire a babysitter to take the kids away- to a movie or something. It is okay to do a reverse babysitting adventure where you just need a little time to be home alone. Just know that you are not the only one who feels like you can't get anything done when everyone is home. I agree. Because YES!

58. Just because something bothers you doesn't mean it bothers anyone else.

The first time I walked to the mailbox of our new home almost two decades ago, I noticed a piece of paper in my driveway. Walking back from the mailbox, I realized that if I did not pick up that paper, nobody else would. I picked up the paper and threw it away. Since then, I have realized that I cannot stand trash in the yard. It doesn't seem to bother anyone else, but it bothers me. Also, I'm not too fond of dust on the glass TV stand, dog hair under the table, bathroom trash being full, empty toilet paper rolls, closing cabinet doors, turning off lamps, or anything else that inadvertently drives me nuts but doesn't seem to bother anyone else. I'm not even sure if my family knows how OCD I am because I do things without saying a word. It's not a big deal, but if I griped about every little thing, that's all I would be doing. Some things really bother me and nobody else. You have two choices: deal with it or don't. If it bothers you that bad, nicely encourage your family or colleagues or whoever to respect the space. If it really isn't that big of a deal, fix it and don't complain. Pick the paper out of the yard. Close the cabinets. Change the toilet paper. Save the nagging or the fussing for something that really matters- like picking up wet swimsuits off the bathroom floor. Now, that is something to fuss about. Because YES!

59. Share your sparkle.

When I started working at a new elementary school a few years ago, it was apparent that the teachers were very glittery. Glitter, Pinterest, cute clothes, decorated rooms, and fancy fonts were just part of the culture. Oh my. Me? I could care less what I wear, and glitter is not my style. But that didn't mean I had a free pass. The first thing that happened was the principal gave me a t-shirt with glittered letters to say, "Welcome!" Oh. My. Gosh. I had a glittered, V-neck, t-shirt that even had a glitter heart on it. Heaven help me. But I wore the dang shirt and eventually found some earrings with just as much sparkle. Before I knew it, I was sparkling more often than not. I found myself using a Cricut machine and designing gorgeous displays and doing all the things. I, too, had learned to sparkle. It's still not really me, but I admit that I kind of feel a little fancy when I'm wearing my trendy shirts and cute earrings. I've learned that when we share our sparkle, it is contagious. So, just embrace the glitter, sparkle a little, and share your sparkle with others. Because YES!

60. Sing when it's funky.

My uncle had a karaoke business many years ago. My husband spent hours and hours learning from Uncle Roy how to build our library to over 10,000 songs. We now have a professional karaoke machine and the professional books with pages and pages full of songs by title and by artist. Did I mention that I am a terrible singer? When I was little, my mom didn't really even want me to sing "Happy Birthday" at parties. Nonetheless, I like to sing in my barn. There's nobody listening (except the neighbors) and it doesn't matter how bad you sound if the music is loud enough. It's okay to be in a funk once in a while. We all get that way. My advice is to find a karaoke machine or just pull up songs on your phone and sing. I suggest Brown Eyed Girl, Under the Boardwalk, Jesse's Girl, New Age Girl, and You've Got The Right Stuff. Just sing. Let it all out. Turn up the volume so you don't hear just how bad you are and sing when it's funky. Because YES!

61. Pond scum means you're in the pond.

My middle child, Danielle, loves live theatre. She has known for years that she loves the film/ movie industry and has recently decided that she wants to make a career working in live theatre. She doesn't want to act on stage, but she likes the technical part of the shows. Regardless of film/ movie/ theatre genre, they all involve public relations and audiences. She has started volunteering and working at different venues to gain experience and exposure. Most recently, she was a camp counselor for a local children's theatre. She volunteered for the camp and ended up getting to be part of the stage crew. The kids put on the play, "Elf" on four different showings and each time, my daughter came out on stage after the play and swept the floor from the fake snow that had fallen. Our family went to each show and stayed after to cheer for her as she did her job. It was wonderful. We were obnoxious the first time and then we tried to be more discreet as the shows went on. The point is that she wasn't just working the play, she was on stage as part of the stage crew. She has since served on many crews and we are just as proud of her as is if she were the main character. She works hard. Sweeping the floor is part of being in the pond. She might be pond scum this production, but next production, she may have the opportunity to run lighting or sound. Each little part is important. You should always do your job to the best of your ability. After all, if you are pond scum, you're still in the pond. Because YES!

62. It IS your job.

To go along with the pond scum YESism, I want to talk about the idea that something is not your job. That drives me crazy. If you are part of something, it IS your job. A few years ago, I was volunteering at my church's Vacation Bible School. One of the light bulbs was out in the room that I was teaching in. I changed it. The janitor said, "I can do that." Nope. I am perfectly capable of changing a light bulb. At a different Vacation Bible School, I had just finished my doctorate degree. I had gone on a little break and went to the bathroom. A kid had smeared poop all over the toilet seat (probably because there was no toilet paper in the stall). I went to find the janitor, but he wasn't there. The preacher and I went to the supply closet and found toilet paper, but we had the task of cleaning the toilet. I volunteered. It was absolutely my job in the moment. We joked about how I have special qualifications as a doctor to handle such incidents. Whatever. The truth is we all have special qualifications regardless of our status, degree, etc... You are never too good to wipe poop off the toilet or change a light bulb. You just aren't. Neither am I. It IS our job. Because YES!

63. Inconvenience is far from a problem.

Man, I can't stand waiting in the pick-up lines at the schools my kids attend. Talk about inconvenience. But, guess what? It is not a problem. There is a difference. Problems have solutions and inconveniences are just that. It is important to know the difference because sometimes we try to solve things that don't have good solutions. You may not like standing in line at the grocery store, but don't be rude about it. It is not a problem, just an inconvenience. If it were really a problem, you probably didn't have time to be there in the first place- which is the problem. If someone messes up your order at a restaurant, that is super frustrating, but in reality, it is not a problem, it is more of an inconvenience. Unless, of course, you are really hungry- then it could be more of a problem, but really, there is an easy solution thus making it more inconvenient than anything. Be nice to people. Know the difference between problems and inconveniences. If there's a problem, try to be a part of the solution. If it is just inconvenience, just try to be patient. Be kind. It's really okay. Because YES!

64. Adult conversations are awesome.

I'm a good mom. I'm actually a really great, all in, almost helicopter-y mom. I am always at my kids' practices and games. I'm involved in their school functions/ activities, and we are always going somewhere together. We are a tight knit family unit and I'll never apologize for that. However, being all in with my kids has often left me out of adult conversations. I don't go out with the girls after work. My husband doesn't meet the guys for a drink after work, either. The problem with being all in is that you forget to be an adult. My husband and I never really go on dates, and that is not healthy. In the last few years, we've been more conscious of making an effort to go out by ourselves. The kids are older and can be left alone for a little bit. Remember the seasons? I have also made a conscious effort to do things with adult women. I participate in an annual girlfriend's sleepover at Christmas time. It is fun. I also attend weekly Toastmaster's meetings with adults. I enjoy an hour a week of adult only conversation. You may not be in a season of opportunity to have adult conversations, but try. Try to make time to just be an adult. Go on a date with your partner. Talk about adult things on purpose. Because YES!

65. Rules and procedures are important. Understanding why we need them is important, too.

In America, we drive on the right side of the road. In our elementary schools, we walk in a straight line on the right side of the hall. We keep our hands by our side and our mouths quiet. We walk in an orderly fashion. Why? Why do we do that? For one, we begin teaching students directionality. You walk on the right side of the hallway because when you get to be an adult, you need to know what side of the road to drive on. We keep our hands to ourselves because we respect personal space. We keep our mouths shut because in elementary school, classes are simultaneously conducting business while others are transitioning. It is important to respect the learning environment. In upper grades, students have passing periods, but that isn't true in elementary. So, that's why we walk silently on the right side of the hall with our hands to ourselves. It shouldn't be a secret, though. Rules are designed to keep people safe and to provide equity in various situations. There are reasons why the rules exist. If you don't like a rule, you don't have permission to break it. You do, however, have the ability to understand and question the rules. I know this all too well. I haven't always been the best rule follower, but I am more apt to follow the rules if I understand why they are there. Because YES!

66. Be old-fashioned and new wave at the same time.

Guilty. I have so many examples for this YESism. For instance, I believe in chivalry and girl power! I love when my husband opens my door, but I can most certainly open my own. I like the church praise band and singing from a hymnal with accompaniment from the piano player. My husband saves parts of things instead of throwing things away. He knows how to fix things. He and his dad would go to the library and look up car parts and engine fixes when he was little. My husband still fixes things, but he's learned to look up YouTube videos that show you how to fix something. He's teaching our kids how to change their tires, fix a toilet, and grill out on their own. It is old-fashioned to save in today's throwaway society. Taking care of our things and fixing what we have might seem old-fashioned in today's fast paced expectations. Just remember that it is okay to be both. Stay true to yourself and respect the old-fashioned ways but be open to growing and learning today. Because YES!

67. Be careful when you are texting with your professor.

In fact, be careful when texting with anyone. The incident that I am thinking about happened a few months ago when one of my adult college students was texting me about an upcoming assignment. I received a "Hurry home. I'm hot for you!" message from the student. The .gif was absolutely inappropriate communication between a student and professor. I simply texted back a question mark and quickly got an apology text. I'm sure the student was more embarrassed than I. Know with whom you are texting. And, do not assume you know just because of the number you are texting. You never know who is on the other end of the line. Furthermore, never send something you wouldn't want your pastor to see. That's the rule of thumb I live by and have tried to teach my kids. You think you are just sending your picture to someone, but once it leaves your phone, you cannot control where it goes. You do not have control once you hit send. You cannot take back what is out there in cyberspace. Just because you delete something does not mean that others have erased it. They may not share it with anyone, but you cannot ever be sure. When I was younger, I went to the mall with some friends. I bought a dress that was skintight and way too short. My mom made me try it on for her, and then as soon as I took it off, she grabbed it and made me clean the toilets with it. She said that if I wanted to look like a tramp, I might as well get used to cleaning toilets-because that is the kind of future I was up against. I asked her how I knew what was okay to wear. She said, "If you have to ask, you already know the answer." That has been such truth in my life. If you have to ask if it is okay to wear something, you probably shouldn't wear it. If you have to think about whether a text is appropriate, it probably isn't. Because YES!

68. Admit when you fail.

Raising teenagers is a whole new season. Sometimes I wish my kids came with instruction manuals. There is no such thing and even the best parenting advice magazines and books cannot prepare you for these years. I have been guilty of reacting in both rational and irrational ways to situations. There are times when I have been absolutely more irrational and reactive than helpful and encouraging as a parent. On more than one occasion, I've had to admit that I was wrong. I think it is important to own up to our mistakes and to admit when we've failed. You can fix most anything in life if you just own up to it. On our last camping trip, Holly backed into a guy's truck that was parked next to us. She hit his cattle guard and didn't even put a scratch on it. She was so upset, though, and didn't know what to do. I put on my shoes and walked over to the guy's trailer, knocked on the door, and let her tell him. Tearfully, she told him she hit his truck and he said, "Calm down. It's just a truck." Then, he put on his shoes and came out. There was absolutely no damage and he looked at her completely dumbfounded. He said, "Are you sure you hit it?" She admitted that she felt the bump but was so sorry. He gave her a hug and told her, "Thank you for being so responsible." No harm, no foul. Just own it. In life, just admit when you make a mistake. Usually, there can be a fix if you just admit when you have made a mistake or overreacted or whatever it is, just admit when you're wrong. Be better tomorrow than you were today. Give yourself grace. Because YES!

69. Do what you say.

I am obsessed with being a person you can count on. If I agree to do something, I will do it. The one thing you can count on me for is my word. I'm not sure there is more to say for this YESism. If people cannot count on you to keep your word, you lack trust and integrity. For those reasons alone, you should always do what you say. Dot. End. Period. Because YES!

70. Dress-up days are fun.

When my son was in kindergarten, I swear they had nine million dress-up days (Tacky tourists, Pilgrims, Grinches, 100th Day of School, 101th Dalmatian Day, etc.). It was expensive and hard to keep up with. But everyone dressed up. Everyone. Here's the deal. If you or your kid is part of an organization or school, and they have dress-up days, try to participate. Seriously. The kids notice. Other people notice. Don't be the parent that doesn't let their kid dress-up unless your kid doesn't want to dress-up. Be creative. If you are a person who coordinates dress-up days, try to keep it simple for everyone. Be aware of how many times you insist that everyone dresses like a pirate, dalmatian, or tacky tourist. Give yourself permission to participate, too! After all, if you are going to dress like a pirate, you might as well add ARR to the end of every sentence all day long. Because YES!

71. Find joy in simplicity.

Many people make a big deal out of making a "bucket list" or a "life list." Some people spend forever trying to figure out what they enjoy. My advice is to keep it simple. Sure, I want to stay in a bungalow in the Galapagos Islands, but I also want to sip coffee uninterrupted on my porch swing. I enjoy watching the birds in my makeshift bird hotel. I enjoy making a fire in the fireplace when it's cold, and I love opening the windows on a brisk spring morning. I enjoy looking at my blankets folded nicely on my quilt rack and the smell of a fresh box of dryer sheets. Think in simple terms when you ponder the things you enjoy. Do you enjoy seeing your clothes on matching hangers? Then buy matching hangers. Do you like the dog being fluffy and smelling good? Then spend time bathing it. Put your life in slow motion by taking a hard look at where and how you spend your time. What do you really value? What are the little things you would miss the most if you never got to do them again? I would be so sad if my porch swing broke. I could possibly die if my coffee pot quit. Slow it down a bit and really think about the things you enjoy and do those more. Keep it simple. Because YES!

72. Make the call.

When my grandmother passed away years ago, I was so thankful that I had saved her last message on my phone. I played her message over and over. I remember her vividly saying, "Good morning, Sunshine! I hope you have a good day. Call me when you can." Dadgum. I can still hear her in my mind. I called her almost every day. She was my hero, and I'd give anything to hear her voice again. My grandmother's best friend is still alive, though, and I talk to her often. I love hearing her voice. I might not have a long time to chat, but I make the call anyway. I implore you to make it a point to take ten minutes and call the people you love. Tell them you love them and you are thinking of them. Seriously. Make the call. Today. Right now. Because YES!

73. Have the best day ever.

SpongeBob sings a song called "The Best Day Ever!" It is goofy. And, not. Why not have the best day ever? You may not have a lot of great stuff going on today, but why can't you have a great day in your situation? A few weeks ago, I had a total hysterectomy. I was in the hospital, and I knew several people were expecting an update. Nobody ever wants to have surgery where they are removing body parts. But my surgery went off without any complications or side effects from anesthesia. I woke up, had some good drugs, and went back to sleep. Later, a respiratory therapist came in to check on me because my oxygen levels kept going down. She said, "Hey! I know you! You were my teacher!" Yes! The professional taking care of me in the hospital was my former fourth grade student. Heck yes! She hugged me, and we had a great conversation. She showed me pictures of her little girl, and it was terrific. My daughter brought Panda Express up to the hospital, and we enjoyed talking and spending the evening together. It was a really great day. Sure, it would have been way more fun to be on a beach somewhere, but with everything taken into consideration, it was a great day. Why have a horrible day? Why not have a great day even though it is difficult? Decide right now that today is the best day ever. If not today, start tomorrow. Every day, try to have a great day. Because YES!

74. You control the narrative.

If we were in person and you were at one of my Perspective Workshops, you might hear me tell the story of being stopped by the police for speeding on the way home from my mom's house. First, I would tell you that a cop had the audacity to pull me over for speeding when I wasn't really even going that fast. He rudely said, "License and Insurance." He didn't even say, "Please." So rude. Then, he went to his car with his lights flashing, making a scene, and returned with a ticket already printed out. No discussion, no warning, just a ticket. So stinking rude. At this point in the workshop, I would take a breath and change the narrative to reflect a different perspective. My story changes to: You'll never believe what a terrific opportunity I had coming home from my mother's house. This faithful public servant pulled me over to remind me of the importance of following the rules. He requested my personal documents so that he could verify my identity and did not waste my time. He simply wrote me a ticket and had it ready quickly so that I could get back on the road. He kept his lights on so that everyone would know that I was on the side of the road, which kept us both safe for the lesson. I got to talk to my kids about respect for the speed limit and show the girls how to behave when being pulled over. Yay! See the difference? You get to control the narrative of every event in your life. You can be mad, and you can be sad, and you can be glad. The only real difference is how you tell the story. The world is not against you. You can make it seem that way by repeating the events of your life in whatever narrative you choose. Your thoughts become your words, your words become your beliefs, and your beliefs form your reality. Choose your narrative wisely. Because YES!

75. Invest in others.

This YESism is inspired by the shepherd who will abandon a flock of sheep to look for the one lost sheep. Every little lamb matters. One of the greatest fears we can fuel is the fear of not mattering to people. Do people really see us? For that reason, I encourage each of us to invest in others. Listen. Really listen. Listen to the people who take the time to talk to you. What are they saying? What are they not saying? Even if it's a quick conversation in the grocery store, try to listen as though you don't have a million other things to think about. For some people, the thing that they really want is for you to just listen to them. That doesn't cost money, but it is an investment in their life. Those investments pay dividends at the weirdest times. You might never see the impact of your kindness, but that doesn't mean that the person doesn't pay it forward. Then again, on several occasions, the kindness I have paid forward has come back exponentially by strangers- or those whom I might not have even realized I touched during some other season of my life. So, take the time to invest in others. Sometimes those investments truly are as easy as taking a minute to listen. Really listen. Because YES!

76. Do a project. Take back your life one corner at a time.

There is a picture that completely depicts my life right this second. On the left side of the picture, there are a bunch of circles that are colored in. On the right side are the same circles except those circles are connected. For me, this book has been making some of those circles connect. I ran a Facebook group for a year while crafting this book. These YESisms were shared and discussed long before they became compiled in this book. Meanwhile, I finished my doctoral degree. I lost weight. I crafted my website and paid for a brand design. One of the last things that I had to do was to get myself ready for whatever is next. I had no real place to work. I defended my dissertation at my kitchen table. I put my laptop on a pack of paper towels so that it was taller and didn't have a reflection in the background. I just kept shifting around until I finally decided to do a project. I carved out a corner of an old feed barn to use as my workspace. That barn has been everything from a kid's clubhouse, to my pickin' barn when I was junking, to a catch-all junk room. I decided that I needed a place to work and host online meetings. I painted the back wall and hung shelving. I put up new curtains over the shelves and erected a card table to hold my computer. I shopped at Hobby Lobby for just the right decorations. Now, I have a beautiful space to use as my background for online activities. My son got me a computer stand and a wireless mouse and keyboard. My middle daughter also moved into the other half of the space to do her Cricut work, and we use one corner for show tack. But, if you meet with me via Zoom, I have a corner that is beautiful, professional, and functional. Carve out a corner of space to host your meetings, work on your hobby, or just read. Whatever you enjoy doing, design your space and do the projects needed to make it functional, beautiful, and enjoyable. Because YES!

77. Pray for others.

I have no problem praying. I pray every morning, and usually, I pray several times a day. I like when people ask specifically for prayers for themselves or their loved ones. It is an honor to pray for others. In his book, "Tacos and Chocolate," Drew Myres talks about praying like Mr. Rogers. Mr. Rogers would make a list of people he was praying for and would intentionally pray for them during his nightly prayer. The problem I have with this is that I am usually worthless after 5 p.m. I have tried praying before bed, and I usually end up falling asleep without finishing. On more than one occasion, I have awakened saying, "Amen." God deserves better from me than falling asleep. If I know someone needs prayer, I stop what I am doing and immediately lift them before the Father. It doesn't have to be a long and drawn-out prayer. God already knows the situation. Instead, I ask for blessings and discernment for the person/ family I am praying for. Decide what and how you'll pray for others. It is important that we take care of each other. There will be a time when you'll need prayers. You need prayer warriors who genuinely want the Father to rain blessings upon you. So, be that person. Be the person who does indeed pray for others. You'll be surprised just how far your prayers can reach. Because YES!

78. Handwritten Thank You notes are the best!

This gets its own YESism. I've already talked about being old-fashioned and new wave at the same time. There are many ways to say "Thank you" that don't require thank you cards and postage. But, if someone takes the time and spends the money to do something nice for you, send them a thank you note. Hand write the person a personal message of gratitude. It will bless you and them. Another exercise I do while leading in-person workshops is to have participants write thank you notes to someone who has wronged them. Once, I had a lady write a thank you note to American Airlines for losing her luggage. She discussed having the opportunity to wear her mom's clothes for a few days since she was visiting her from out of state. They were able to take lots of pictures wearing those clothes, and she looked just like her mom. The woman's mom had passed when we did the letter-writing exercise. She wrote about the blessing that came from the lost luggage despite the stress it caused. She then expressed how much fun she had replacing all the lost clothes. It was a handwritten note that she had no intention of ever sending, but it was fun to thank someone for the lessons learned. I encourage everyone to write out thank you notes to people, places, and even situations. Some are fun to mail; others are just to help you let go of the anger and frustration you may feel toward a person or situation. Take a few minutes and handwrite a thank-you note today. Because YES!

79. Challenge someone and challenge yourself.

As young Christians, we were challenged to have accountability partners. In athletics, we were encouraged to have workout partners. I'm always looking for a buddy, partner, or friend. I encourage you to find a friend who will push you to do great things. I have a few friends from different walks of life who encourage and push me to be better today than I was yesterday. They are gems. These women are not jealous, judgmental, and they have no investment in my success- except to be happy for me. The same is true on my end. I do not understand why we can't all be happy for one another. If I see another person experiencing success and doing great things, I'm the first to offer a high five and congratulations! Look for ways to build up another person. The world will provide enough reasons for us to fail or feel defeated. To combat the negative Nellies, I suggest you find someone with the same goals, aspirations, and dreams. Encourage them every single day. The encouragement you'll receive will be twice as much as you give. That is a consequence of the Universe. By increasing the goodness and encouragement you put into the Universe, the Universe responds with just as much, if not more, energy than you can imagine. So the challenge is to encourage someone and find someone who challenges you! Because YES!

80. Life isn't always sunshine and rainbows. Dance anyway.

Happiness is a choice every single day. We don't always get to choose our situation, but we control how we respond. Am I grateful? Yes. Always. Am I happy? Yes. Mostly. Am I positive? I'm working on it. For two decades, my children have faced unbelievable circumstances, and we've been in and out of the hospital. Last night, Scottish Rite called, and it's time for our annual check-up. Dang. That also means it's time for Taylin's cardiologist check-up. Dang. And the neurologist check-up for Dani- Dang. And Endocrine on Friday for Holly. Dang. I am learning to make conscious choices to be happy despite my situation. I consider it a learned behavior and a way to increase my overall joy in life. I know I try to be PollyAnna, and YES! most of the time these days. I still struggle sometimes to live in the YES! of every day like I struggle to stay on Keto. I like cheeseburgers with buns and onion rings. Actually, I like onion rings a lot, but I have to choose what I allow into my body to meet my weight goals. The same is true with happiness. It is easy to go down a rabbit hole or stay upset or live in constant fear. I sure don't like the looming appointments already on the calendar, but I'm not going to think about the what-ifs. Don't get me wrong—my kids struggle. My kids make choices I disagree with. My kids act like fools, make messes, act entitled, think they can talk back to me, leave their dishes in their rooms, towels on the floor, and say things to each other that break my heart. But, they also love fiercely, talk constantly, play games, go places, and tell each other they "love you more." If I let myself, I could focus only on what they do wrong... what a tragedy that would be, though, because I might miss out on so many more terrific things they do right. Saying YES! and choosing to be happy is a much better option than the stress, doubt, fear, depression, anxiety, and grief that I was living in. Like my desire to eat onion rings, sometimes I must fight hard not to partake in those feelings. It seems weird but learning to choose Joy has been a process for me. It doesn't mean that I am perfect, without problems, without fear, worry, doubt, etc; it just means that I am making a conscious choice to be happy. I still don't have a ton of money yet- but I'm learning to live in affluence (plenty). We still get sick and have medical things, but I choose to think about wellness. I still get my feelings hurt, but I try to let it go. I'm not happy all the time, but I'm happier than I was. I'm not skinny, but I'm thinner than I was. Every single day, I choose to increase my joy through gratitude and awareness of potentiality. I'm attempting to inspire and empower others to do the same- because YES! Imagine if we all awakened our joyful, happy selves- what could we accomplish together? It isn't always sunshine and rainbows, but I'm happier than I have ever been as an adult, by choice. I get to decide today to focus on happiness, and I encourage you to do the same. Do something today that brings you joy. Remember that life isn't always sunshine and rainbows. Dance anyway. On purpose. Because YES!

81. Disconnect and unplug occasionally. It won't kill you.

Take a break. Leave your phone turned off for five minutes. When you survive those five minutes, leave it off for another ten minutes. Then, creep up to an hour. When you figure out that you haven't needed your phone for an hour, stretch out the time for a few hours. Work up to the point of not using your phone (or tablet, computer, watch) for a whole day. You are not alone. I am addicted to my phone, but I have also learned to let it go. You do not have to answer every single text or social media post. There used to be a time when these devices did not exist, and our ancestors survived. You will survive. Try to go a whole day without television. What? A full day without Roku, Hulu, Netflix, Prime, or Fubo? YES! A whole day- or two- or seven. Take a step back and let your eyes rest. Let your brain rest. Just like an addict feels disconnected without another hit, or an alcoholic craves another drink, we have become so addicted to our phones that we wear them. We have ear pods and watches that ding from our phones. Where does it end? Where do you fit into to your own connectivity? Are you having facetime with the people in your life? Real facetime. If not, then throw your phone in the toilet. If you spend more time searching and scrolling and watching TikTok, STOP IT. If all your inspiration comes from Pinterest, STOP IT. If you only know what your family is doing because of Facebook posts, STOP IT. If you only know how to date and break up with someone via text, STOP IT. Unplug. Give your mind, body, and soul permission to connect for real, in real life. Have real, uninterrupted, intentional conversations. Give yourself time to think without being distracted by a notification. And, don't be kind-of unplugged. You know, where you only "check" your phone every time you walk by. No. Stop it. Turn off your phone intentionally- especially at the dinner table. What? You don't eat at the table? Stop. Turn off your phone and share a meal without your phones. At least every once in a while. And, by the way, this YESism is a reminder for myself. Because YES!

82. Do the work.

After my daughter's back injury, I suffered from depression, anxiety, and what I have self-diagnosed as Post Traumatic Stress Disorder. My panic attacks were rampant, and I couldn't shake the feeling of despair and fear. I might not have ever thrown a bomb in Iraq, but the sense of impending doom was certainly my reality. Every time my phone rang, I just knew someone was in the hospital. Every time we went to the doctor, I packed a bag with a toothbrush and a pair of socks. Who am I kidding? I kept my hospital bag in my car. I started keeping a hospital bag packed when Holly had her pneumococcal infections, Dani had her asthma admissions, and Taylin had his spinal surgeries. I became better about being more intentional with what I kept in the car in case something terrible happened in the middle of the night. But after Holly's back injury, I went into a total tailspin of doom and gloom. I wouldn't let the gas in my car go below ¾ of a tank in case we had to get to the hospital. I quit answering my phone and texts asking us how we were doing. It was embarrassing. I couldn't stop crying. No matter how many times I posted updates or tried to spin my narrative, I just couldn't stop thinking and feeling overwhelmed, nervous, and scared. I was afraid to be optimistic because the letdown was inevitable. I was out of control. I started wanting to feel better and decided to go to counseling. I'm cheap, so I chose a counseling center through a local church. I figured I needed God, too, so it was a perfect choice. I remember the counselor letting me talk for an hour a week and I cried more than I talked. She kept telling me we were going to do the work, but we had to get to a point where we could start doing the work. I am a doer. I like solutions. Just tell me what the work is, and it will get done. It wasn't that easy, though. I had to dig through about six weeks of word vomit to figure out that I was crying less and able to communicate my fears. Then, we began infusing little tasks, and eventually, I got better. I'm not perfect, and the PTSD comes back at the strangest times, but I have learned new neuropathways to combat the fears. I've started to create a "Do the Work" type of self-help therapy plan that should be ready by the time this book is in publication. Maybe my experience and twist on traditional counseling can help you. Maybe you need a professional as I did. Maybe you have no idea what I'm talking about. I hope you don't. But, for some of you reading this book, know that overwhelming fear, anxiety, panic, and nervousness do not have to define you. It may be where you are, but you can find ways back to happiness on purpose. Yes, there is work, but we are all a work in progress. Do the work. Because YES!

83. Teach a man to fish.

Fishing is my most favorite thing in the world to do. I love fishing, but it has never been about the fish. I love the time with my dad. For the longest time, it was just me and my dad who went fishing. We'd go early in the morning and get back around noon. It was our special time to talk since the private lake we fish in is over an hour from our house. My son has been bitten by the fishing bug. For him, it is more about the fish. I love watching my dad teach my son to fish. Casting, choosing your bait, tying the knot, taking the fish off the hook, and my favorite, kissing the fish for luck. I love those people. I know the saying is, "Give a man a fish, and he'll be hungry tomorrow. Teach a man to fish, and he'll never be hungry again." For all purposes, teaching someone a craft or trade of any kind helps them learn life skills for the future. For me, though, teaching a man to fish is more about recognizing the value of time. Sure, we watch the weather and the wind speed, the ripples on the water, and the way that fish seem to bite when the sun barely starts to breach the horizon. Those are all part of the lessons, but being present, still, and listening to each other is really the investment. Learning to fish is an important skill but learning to spend time together and making time for each other is the real lesson. Whatever it is that you enjoy doing, teach a man (or woman) how to enjoy it, too. Because YES!

84. If you want something, ask for it.

We've talked about saying what you want out loud, but let's talk about asking for what we want. My oldest daughter has a heart of pure gold. I remember taking her to a flea market once. We told her she could have anything she wanted if she'd just ask. We went up and down every aisle and stopped at almost every vendor. She'd look and look but would never ask for anything. We kept trying to get her to ask us, but she wouldn't. Finally, on the way to the car, she stopped at the very last vendor. They had a horse in a purse for five dollars. She held it up and batted her long brown eyelashes at my husband. He said, "Ask me for it." She put it down and we walked to the car. We just about got out of the parking lot, and she said, "Daddy, can I have the horse?" Of course, we turned around and went back, parked, got out of the car and walked her back to the table, and bought the horse. She finally asked. Thank goodness. She did this again in the mall. We were in a dollar store. We were about to leave because she couldn't decide on anything. On the way out of the store, she grabbed a toilet plunger and said, "Can I have this?" We told her she could have anything she asked for, so guess what? We bought the plunger. I don't have any idea why she chose a plunger, except it was the last thing on the way out of the store. What I do remember is that for the rest of the mall trip, she used the plunger almost like a walking stick. Plop, suck, pull. Plop, suck, pull. All through the mall. It was so embarrassing!! But she asked for it. Finally! I think that a lot of the time, we don't get something because we don't ask for it. We can't decide what we want, so we settle for a toilet plunger. If we would just ask, I bet we'd get more of what we want. One of the times we were in the hospital, I jokingly asked the nurse if there was a laundry mat there. My blanket and clothes were smelling awfully hospital-ly. Within less than an hour, Child Life was in my hospital room with Tide pods and fabric softener. They told me that the parent laundry room was literally four doors down and offered to stay with my kid while I started a load. ARE YOU SERIOUS? All of the hospital stays and dirty laundry that I've dealt with, and there was literally a parent laundry room on our hospital floor? Yes! All you have to do is ask. Everything you want and need in this life already exists. Read that again. All the money in the world already exists. All of the places you want to visit already exist. Everything is energy. Your job is to connect your desires to whatever you desire. Matthew 7:7-8 says, "Ask, and it shall be given you; seek, and ye shall find; knock, and it shall be opened unto you: For every one that asketh receiveth; and he that seeketh findeth; and to him that knocketh it shall be opened." Now, I believe that in context, the Bible is referencing spiritual wisdom and the idea that when you search for God, He will reveal himself to you. Out of context, though, the passage is still powerful. This reminds me of the idea that you will miss all the shots you never took in a basketball game. If you never take the shot, you will never score. What is the worst that can happen? You miss? What about asking for something? If you have to ask, you didn't have it in the first place. If you ask and are told no, it's okay. No harm, no foul. You never really know what the answer is going to be, so just ask. Ask for what you want and expect the answer to be YES! Because YES!

85. No regrets. Have a piece of pie- but take a walk.

Dieting is not hard. Who am I kidding? Dieting is hard for people like me who love food. I am a social eater. When I want to go somewhere, I think about what we'll eat while we're out. I plan my meals around what we are doing as a family, but I think about the food as much as I think about the activities. Maybe it is just part of my role as a Mom, but food is a part of my daily life. I lost a large amount of weight on the Keto diet. I don't particularly love the diet, but I do appreciate what it did for me. It worked. No surgery, no meal plan, just meats and fats. Whatever. Now that I am maintaining, though, I find that I allow myself to have things in moderation. If I want a piece of pie, I eat it. But, instead of just eating pie, I eat as little crust as I can and then take a walk. I try to make good choices and balance my eating with movement. I'll skip the potatoes, but I might have a small helping of ice cream occasionally. It's okay. No regrets. You can't change what has already happened, so try to make better decisions next time. If you know you're going to decide to eat a treat (like eating ice cream), simply make a plan to incorporate more exercise. Buy the fancy Michael Kors purse you want but make it a point to eat at home for two weeks instead of going out (and actually eat the leftovers for lunch). I can't remember how many times I didn't go somewhere or do something because I didn't have the money. Not anymore. I just figure it out. I do not deprive myself of a hot fudge sundae, but I may not eat one single carb for three days after. I might fast for 24 hours or more if I overindulge. Whatever it is that you do, own the decision. The only person you need to justify anything to is yourself. Try to make good decisions and live freely but find the balance that helps you live without regrets. Spend the money, eat the pie, whatever it is, just find ways to make more good decisions than bad and own them. Take a walk and be better tomorrow than you were today. Because YES!

86. It doesn't have to be hard.

People complicate things all the time. Myself included. There is an excuse and a reason for life to be hard. But, life doesn't have to be hard. You don't have to be broke. You don't have to be sad. You don't have to be lonely. You don't have to be less. You might feel that things aren't going your way, and they might not be. Not once have my different life domains lined up in perfect harmony. Something always has the potential to blow up in my face, but life in general does not have to be hard. Figure out ways to live in abundance and to choose happiness. If you are struggling with relationships, start being thankful for the people present in your life. If you are struggling with finances, start being thankful for the money you do have. If you are struggling with addiction, be thankful for the choices available to combat it. Life can be hard, but it doesn't have to be. We can and should make better choices that lead to more of what we enjoy. We might not be able to change the exact situation we are in now, but we can start to shift our energy toward what we want. We can take ownership of our lives and start twisting the narrative to complement our future selves. After all, if we were just supposed to be born, pay bills and die, what would be the point? Aren't we supposed to live happily ever after? I sure hope so! It doesn't have to be hard. Choose YES. Because YES!

87. Someone is watching.

Even as I write this book, my kids are watching. I've been talking about this book for a long time. If I don't finish it, I not only let myself down, but I also let them down. You should finish what you start. Whatever you are doing, your kids are watching. Even if you don't have kids, someone is watching and taking their cues from you. I could give us a thousand reasons why we need to make good choices, watch our language, and be kind. One of the most significant reasons, though, is someone is watching you, looking up to you, and making judgments about their own life by comparing themselves to you. In some form or fashion, we observe others and reflect on our own behaviors. "Judgement" may be too harsh of a word, but ultimately, our actions or lack of action influences others. I want my kids to grow up knowing that working hard is not an option- it is an expectation. I don't want them to know how we have and continue to struggle amidst the hospital bills and living the lifestyle we do, but I want them to see that when you work hard, there are rewards. I want my kids to know that they CAN go to school and earn their degrees. I want them to know that there is nothing more important to me than spending time with them. I want them to take risks, be intentional, be honest, be humble and know who they are to the core. How can I teach them that, though, if I am scared or stuck in a life that does not reflect my true self? How can I teach them to live freely if I am bound? How can I teach them to be kind and help others if I never volunteer? What do our everyday actions teach our kids? Do we yield to expectations and social norms? Do you want your kids to live with reservations, to be unintentional with their spending habits, to haphazardly waste their precious time, or to live in lack? I don't. I want my kids to choose adventure, to live on purpose, and to intentionally seek joy and do things they enjoy. Remember that someone is watching you, your choices, and your actions. Who do you want them to see? Because YES!

88. Enough is abundance for most.

In recent months, I have studied my relationship with money. I've come to learn that an affluent lifestyle has nothing to do with your bank account. I would love to know what it feels like to have a maid and a closet with a mirror, but that does not define living with abundance. I have excellent relationships with my family, and I am able to do most of the things I want to do. I might not be able to book a fancy destination vacation yet, but I can book a weekend down in Galveston on the beach. That is enough. Taking my family to the beach for a weekend is the dream of many other families. For those reasons, I live in abundance. Try to look at areas in your life where you have enough. How does that feel? Be thankful for what you do have and start to realize that you are enough. You working on yourself is enough. Everything you dream of already exists, and you can have it all. Your job is to recognize and appreciate what you do have. Grow through gratitude and begin to celebrate who you are, right now. Quit thinking about what you don't have because negativity attracts more negativity. The Universe responds to what we put out there, so if you are only thinking about what you can't afford, you don't allow yourself to be able to afford things. Start thinking about how much you can afford- even if it is just a few gallons of gas. Tell yourself, "I am worthy of this gas. I am thankful for the money to be able to put gas in my car. I am thankful for a job to be able to drive to. I am thankful for the people who work to keep this gas pump working. I am thankful for this car that makes it possible for me to get to work. I am thankful to be healthy enough to pump my own gas and to be able to pay for it." It may seem silly, but changing your attitude helps shift yourself into a different realm of abundance. Quit thinking about what you don't have and be thankful for what you do. You do have enough. When you have enough, you realize you just might be living in abundance. Because YES!

89. Everyone has dirty laundry. Some people just hide it in the closet.

When my father-in-law died, we had the memorial service at our church, and then everyone came back to our home to share a meal. I cleaned and prepped for almost a week. The service was short and sweet. My best friend skipped the service and went to pick up the chicken so it would be hot and fresh for everyone to eat when we got home. Other than that, my mom and I had all the preparations done, and things were laid out. It was easy to finish putting the final touches on the buffet table I had set up. Some people stayed later than others, but eventually, they all left. Our home had been beautifully decorated for the holiday season, and everything was clean. Not fancy, but clean. Dinner was perfect, and we had more than enough food for an army. The next day, however, I got tickled at just how much laundry had piled up in my closet. For a whole week, the focus was on cleaning the house, finishing the Christmas decorations, making the service arrangements, meeting with the funeral home, and cleaning out the apartment where my father-in-law lived. There was much to be done, but oddly enough, laundry never stopped piling up. I spent the whole day washing and folding clothes, towels, blankets, etc. It felt normal, and I began thinking about the clothes in my closet. The whole house was perfectly cleaned. Things were taken care of. Dinner was perfect. To an outsider, we had it all together. What they couldn't see was the pile of laundry almost waist-deep in my closet. It made me think about how we all have dirty laundry. We don't air our dirty laundry for everyone to see, but we all have it. Literally and metaphorically speaking, we all have some form of dirty laundry and secrets from our past. You don't have to disclose what is in your closet. Close the door and let it be. Deal with it when the time is right. You do have to eventually deal with the laundry pile, or you'll run out of clothes or be unable to open your closet door but do it when the time is right. It's okay and perfectly normal to hide that laundry. It would be embarrassing if everyone knew just how much laundry was in the closet- but some things are not for others to know. Guess what, though? Everyone has dirty laundry they may be hiding in a closet. Because YES!

90. Put your hands in the air!

In Laughing Yoga, there is a standard way to greet others. You clap your hands straight up and down and say, "Very good, Very good, YAY!" When you say, "YAY!" You throw your hands in the air in a high V with your palms spread apart, facing away from your body. There is science in this process, even if it sounds crazy. By clapping your hands in the middle of your body, you are connecting your hemispheres and bringing your personal energy to the center. By doing it twice, you reinforce the idea of "very good." When you release the energy into the air and allow yourself to be palms up, open, and extended, you invite the endorphins to magically sprinkle serotonin into your body. Your body has a physiological response to this practice and begins to change you on a molecular level. In my younger days, I would have been rolling my eyes, but it is the truth. Your body is energy. Your mind is the most powerful tool to combat whatever ails you. Neurocognitive restructuring is truly an art form. You can change the trajectory of your future by recognizing just how powerful your thoughts are. You can be happy your whole life without ever attending a laughing yoga class, but why not learn about the science behind something as simple as where to place your hands? Remember that palms up during meditation puts you in a position of receiving. These things have real, physiological effects on your mind, body, and mood. Crossing your arms and frowning can have equally effective consequences at the molecular level. I don't want those consequences, though. Those are energy-sucking, closed off, and far from the abundance that I seek behaviors. If you find that you need a quick pick me up during the day, go to the bathroom and do a "Very good. Very good. YAY!" series. You can do it in public, but people might think you're weird. Try praying and meditating with your palms facing the sky. Put yourself in a position to receive blessings. Little things such as these two little techniques can add up to great results. They surely aren't going to hurt anything- right? And, when you figure out they work, show someone else how to raise their hands in the air! Because YES!

91. Begin with the end in mind.

Your GPS will take you where you want to go, but first, you have to program your destination. Where do you want to end up? Do you remember the Cheshire Cat in Alice in Wonderland? Here is a refresher of the dialogue between the two:

> Alice: Would you tell me, please, which way I ought to go from here?
> Cheshire Cat: That depends a good deal on where you want to get to.
> Alice: I don't much care where.
> Cheshire Cat: Then it doesn't much matter which way you go.

The Cheshire Cat makes the point that if you don't know where you are headed, then it doesn't matter which direction you go. Don't even bother programming your GPS, because without direction, any road will get you there. But, if you want to reach your destination in the shortest route possible, or if you need help staying on track, you've got to focus on where you are headed. Our GPS will fuss at us if we pull over for gas. It will tell us to turn around if we make a wrong turn. It will reroute our plan if we veer off the course. It can only do that, though, if it knows where we intend to end up. The same is true for our lives. My workshop participants complete a mapping exercise where we draw a road that has led us to this exact moment. Our road maps include unique stops along the way. Then, we turn over the paper and draw another road. We think about things we want to happen in the next 10 years. We ask questions, like what "stops" would we want to make? In the next decade, what do you want to do? Where do you want to be in 10 years? How can you begin with the end in mind? How can you accomplish those goals along the way? You can take a detour or change your path- remember, you are the boss. At some point, though, time starts speeding up, and you realize that ten years is but a drop in the bucket. So, where do you want to be? In 10 years, what do you want to have accomplished? How are you going to do it? What is your plan? What obstacles do you need to overcome? What are you going to ask for? Spend some serious time sketching out your plan, and then begin to program your internal GPS. Start to navigate toward a better, more intentional, happier version of yourself. Program your internal GPS by beginning with the end in mind! Because YES!

92. Make a list.

I'm a list girl. I find it funny that I have created a "list husband" and "list kids." My husband is such a good man, but he is easily distracted. He will do just about anything we ask him to do, but he has difficulty staying focused when there is much to be done. My kids are the same way. They will do whatever is on their list. They won't go out of their way to do much more, but if they have a list, they'll work and cross things off as they finish each task. I find that making a list helps our family work toward a common goal. I have all sorts of things on my daily to-do list. I try to write everything down even if I have no intention of doing anything about it that day. I keep a "Later" list on a clipboard on my microwave. When I know that there is something that I can't get done on my to-do list, I transfer it to the "Later" list. I crossed it off today's list because adding it to the "Later" list enabled me to deal with it. I decided to let it go, and then I didn't think about it again until "Later." Sometimes I pull out the "Later" list for review. Most of the time, the things on the "Later" list have taken care of themselves, or they aren't important anymore. Great! I reflect and think, "Gosh, I should have done that." Either way, I know that at the end of the day, I did what I could, and I'm okay with that. Give yourself permission to have and keep a "Later" list. Handle what you can and give yourself permission to cross things off that can be handled later. Because YES!

93. Go for a walk.

Walking shoes have literally saved my marriage and kept me out of prison on more than one occasion. I walk for exercise purposes and for my mental health. When I am trying to find the words to express how frustrated I am with my husband, kids, job, etc. I find that taking a walk can help me gain clarity. I walk by myself and think about how and what to say when I calm down most of the time. Most of the time, no one but me knows that I am irritated beyond irritation. My walking time helps me refocus and breathe while I think about why I am upset. Walking affords me the time I need to think about the situation and how I will deal with it most appropriately- or not. I always wear two sports bras when I go for a walk. I know, TMI, but let me explain. One reason is so that things stay where they are supposed to, and the other reason is so that I can tuck my cell phone into my bra on speakerphone. Sometimes, I can talk out my problems with my mom. Sometimes, I call different friends who are experts that can help me see my options. Sometimes, I just need to listen to a good book with a positive message. That's how I listen/ read so many good self-help books. Other times, I just pray and ask God to intervene. Most of the time, though, when I am back from my walk, I have a good idea of why I'm upset, what I am going to do about it, and how to use my energy in a positive way to change the narrative. It works for me. For me, walking is therapy. There is a walking garden at our local children's hospital. It is a circular garden with a fountain in the middle. You're supposed to cast your cares in prayer on the way in and count your blessings on the way out. I've walked that garden a million times. I find that the practice works on my daily walks, too. I spend the first half of the walk griping, yelling, cussing, or just silently debating. Then on the way back, I try to find solutions and happiness and blessings. Not all walks are profoundly engaging and soul searching. Often, I am just walking to stay in shape. Other times, though, it is about giving myself permission to take a few steps away and think about what is and what I want. If you prefer swimming or boxing or yoga, do that instead of taking a walk. But do something productive and helpful. Make a plan right now that you will stick to the next time you feel icky. You will have problems in the future; we all will. So, decide right now that the next time you are faced with a situation, you'll go for a walk- or something physically engaging and give yourself permission to think. Because YES!

94. Walk outside without shoes.

I remember when my mom made me do this. I was angry and super irritated at her nonsense. She made us take off our shoes and walk outside on the grass. So dumb. But it felt good. The grass felt good. And the sunshine felt great. I am not sure which was the best, but working together, the act of taking off my shoes and walking barefoot on the grass seemed to settle my soul- at least for a few minutes. My husband, not so much. He was irritated that his mother-in-law was bossing him around, and I was letting her. Nonetheless, he obeyed. Pretty soon, we were laughing, and again, I'm not sure if it was the laughter or the grass, but I started to feel better. Walking outside without shoes won't hurt you, and it just might help you feel grounded. Just like laughing, doing yoga, and meditating with your palms facing the sky. The point is to try something new. Be open to new experiences and know that you do have choices. Take a walk outside barefoot. Because YES!

95. Stay in bed an extra 8 minutes.

Don't just wake up. Begin. Start. My alarm clock goes off most days around 4 a.m. I purposely leave my alarm clock just out of arm's reach so that I have to get up to snooze it. I walk to the kitchen to start my coffee and then get back in bed for the next 8 minutes. I usually drift back to sleep for a few minutes. When the snooze goes off again, I silence it and begin praying and visualizing the day. I think about how I will feel at the end of the day. I start thinking about what I can do to make things run smoothly and what I will be intentional about. Then, I pray for my family, friends, and other people in my heart. I go through one more snooze cycle if I'm not done praying. Otherwise, I get up and get going. Since I teach online, I work first, then get ready before I wake up the kids. My routine doesn't change much, even when I do not set the alarm. I still wake up, start the coffee, get back in bed, visualize the day and pray. I am intentional about two things: visualization and prayer. I begin with the end in mind, and I think about how I think the day will go. I might be completely kidding myself, but I at least set my mind on success for the day. Then, I make a point to spend a few minutes talking with the Big Guy. If I waited until the evening, I would forget or fall asleep. I do pray at night, but ultimately my routine reflects morning reverence. Give yourself permission to hit the snooze, but use the 8-minute intervals to prepare your mind for whatever tasks the day presents. Because YES!

96. Tip extra.

When I was in high school, we would go to this fantastic Mexican restaurant and order chips and green and red sauce. Writing about it now makes my mouth water. My friend and I would order water and chips and say we were waiting on our parents. Our parents never showed up and after three baskets of chips and countless bowls of green sauce, we were stuffed. We would leave a dollar or two on the table and apologize for our absent parents. I'm pretty sure they caught onto us at some point, but they never said anything. We were young, broke kids. Looking back, I wish I knew who our servers were because I would go back and pay for all the times I ate for free- literally. As an adult, I try to make it a point to always tip appropriately. Sometimes money is tight, but if you are eating out for dinner or receiving any service, you should budget the tip. It is part of the experience, and the people serving you depend on your generosity. I try to remember that. Now that my kids are older and working, I see how much of a difference it makes. I never really worked in a service industry (unless you count the summers I drove the beer cart at the golf course), but I know that my kids use their money for college. They buy gas, books, Starbucks, and whatever else the college kids need. My oldest works birthday parties at the local gym, and usually, the workers are tipped generously. Receiving generous tips makes her day, and I try to remember that when I am out. Be kind. And, if you're working in a service industry, take care of your people. I tip much better when the service is excellent. I love to see people working hard, and I appreciate your service. Thank you. Let's make an effort to respect those who serve us by tipping extra. Because YES!

97. Be the beginning. Pay it forward.

Speaking of Starbucks, I cannot count the number of times I have inadvertently been the recipient of a pay-it-forward in the drive-through. I keep it going! If you didn't know, if you have your drink paid for you and they said it was part of the pay-it-forward, please pay for the next person. Don't be the broken link. Also, a little game my parents play on vacation is, "Pick the Couple." When we are on vacation, we usually eat breakfast at the hotel, grab a quick lunch, and enjoy a sit-down dinner. At the restaurant, we look around and pick a couple or a family, and we buy their dinner. It is fun to watch them wait for the ticket and realize someone has paid for their meal. Usually, they look around and we all just look away. It's our little secret. I love doing that. I play this same game with my kids now, too! The craziest thing happened a few months ago. We went to a football game at my daughter's college. At the end of the game, the kids decided to order a pizza and stay with her in her dorm room. My husband and I could have gone anywhere in the town to eat, but we went to a cozy little diner and sat at the counter. We laughed. We got to chit-chat with the waitress behind the counter and just had the best time. When it was time to pay, the waitress told us it was already paid for. We looked around and couldn't figure out who to thank, so we just left the waitress a big tip and walked out. It felt so weird. We were the old couple that we usually look for! How crazy is that? Anyway, when you pay it forward, it blesses you and the recipient. And, you just never know when someone is going to pay it forward for you. Be the beginning! Because YES!

98. Introduce yourself.

My kids always ask me if I know a stranger. Nope! I sure don't. Remember in the movie Forrest Gump when Forrest wasn't allowed to talk to or take rides from strangers? He introduced himself to the bus driver, then Dorothy Harris introduced herself. Forrest said, "Well, now we ain't strangers anymore." I think that line has just stuck with me forever. Remember that most people are good. You have just as much right to breathe the air as the next person. We all put our pants on one leg at a time. You cannot be too rich or famous for me. You cannot be too poor or insignificant for me. We are the same. I could care less if you are the Queen of England or the janitor of the hotel where I am staying. You are important. You matter. I'll shake your hand any day of the week. I'll look you in the eyes and introduce myself. We may not appear to have anything in common, but we have more in common than you think. Don't be afraid to introduce yourself. It takes two seconds to not be a stranger anymore- right, Forrest? Because YES!

99. Do things your own way.

Why not 100 YESisms? Because YES! One hundred would be cliché and expected. Are there more YESisms? YES! I'm sure there are. For the sake of wrapping up this adventure, though, I'm going to end at 99. It feels right. Do we always have to follow the rules? I hope by now you've learned that the answer is "hardly." You don't have to do anything you don't want to do. You can choose to give yourself permission to adopt a happier, more enjoyable lifestyle by saying YES! to the things you enjoy. You get to be the author of your own story, and you are responsible for your narrative. For me, I think 99 is a cool number. Because YES!

# EPILOGUE

Here's how I applied Because YES! to a list I made on January 29, 2021, when my middle child was hospitalized with a migraine:

1. Twenty-one adults helped my daughter yesterday. Twenty-one medical professionals were involved in the care of my kid. I'm thankful for each person who chose a life of service, including the security guard who walked me to my car.
2. I'm thankful for modern medicine and diagnostic tests. Knowing what is "not" is as important as knowing what "is." We've ruled out some big, scary things. That's good. Finding exactly what is going on is going to take some time.
3. I'm thankful for hospital beds in private rooms. We even had a private room in the ER. This room we're in now has a bed for Dani and a parent couch that turns into a bed. There is a parent room next door for coffee and ice water. Remote control TV and pillows are available- I do not take that for granted.
4. I'm thankful for a work team that instantly said, "How can we help?" I knew that my students were well taken care of and loved. That means the world to a teacher.
5. I'm thankful for a husband that volunteered to bring me a blanket because I was freezing! I finally asked for one myself, but he would have driven 45 minutes just to make sure I warmed up. That warms my heart. I know my other two kids

are safe, happy, loved, and cared for. My support team is phenomenal.

6. I'm thankful for the broccoli and cheese soup. It wasn't my favorite, but it was warm and was a healthy choice for my diet. I didn't have to break ketosis even though I really could have eaten a horse last night.

7. I'm thankful for children's hospitals. Of course, COVID-19 has things locked down, but it's still a colorful place filled with people who love kids. I love the details in every nook and cranny that scream, "We love kids!"

8. I'm thankful that the meds are working for Dani. The doctor said we may or may not see neurology before we go home, but we should be able to go home this morning. We'll do an outpatient visit if we get discharged before they make rounds.

9. I'm thankful that my lesson plans were ready to post, and all my copies were already prepared. There is joy in planning ahead so that you can allow yourself to be present in the moment.

10. I'm thankful that when I am weak, He is strong.

Because YES!

# Resources

Allen, R. (2008). *Green light classrooms: Teaching techniques that accelerate learning*. Corwin Press.

Bennett, R. T. (2020). *The light in the heart: Inspirational thoughts for living your best life*. Roy T. Bennett.

Byrne, R. (2012). *The magic* (Vol. 3). Simon and Schuster.

Dweck, C. (2014). TED Talk. *The power of yet. Retrieved from https://www. youtube. com/watch.*

King, Jeanie (2019). *Giddy Up, Girl! Why are you waiting?.* Kindle.

Manson, M. (2016). *The Subtle Art of Not Giving a F\* ck: A Counterintuitive Approach to Living a Good Life*. Macmillan Publishers Aus..

McRaven, A. W. H. (2017). *Make Your Bed: Little Things that Can Change Your Life... and Maybe the World*. Hachette UK.

Myers, Drew (2021). *The tacos and chocolate diet: How to live a bold, adventurous, and intentional life*. Open Mouth Media.

Nelson-Schmidt, M. (2012). *Jonathan James and the whatif monster*. Kane Miller.

Pyle, H. (1992). Wisdom's wages and folly's pay.

Sincero, J. (2013). *You are a badass: How to stop doubting your greatness and start living an awesome life*. Running Press Adult.

Tuttle, C. (2018). Mastering affluence: 6 lessons to create a life you love. Live Your Truth Press.

Tuttle, C. (2003). *Remembering Wholeness: A Personal Handbook for Thriving in the 21st Century*. Live Your Truth Press.

# ABOUT THE AUTHOR

Dr. Tina Bernard has been a professional educator for over two decades. She holds a Doctorate in Educational Leadership with an emphasis on Curriculum and Instruction. Dr. Bernard's research has primarily focused on metacognition, critical and creative thinking, neuroplasticity, and improving educator pedagogy. She holds a master's degree in Educational Psychology. She has authored several journal articles and book chapters concerning engaging the learner through motivation and empowerment. While Dr. Bernard is a skillful educational thought leader, she is also an inspirational woman with a personal story of overcoming many obstacles despite the uncanny set of unique circumstances. Dr. Bernard's passion is to encourage others to become the best version of themselves by intentionally choosing to say "YES!"

Made in the USA
Columbia, SC
14 June 2022

61687786R00089